The Herbal Menopause Book

by Amanda McQuade Crawford

 The Crossing Press
Freedom, California

The information contained in this book is based on the experience and research of the author. It is not intended as a substitute for consulting with your physician or other health care provider. Any attempt to diagnose and treat an illness should be done under the direction of a health care professional. The publisher does not advocate the use of any particular health care protocol, but believes that the information in this book should be available to the public. The publisher and author are not responsible for any adverse effects or consequences resulting from the use of any of the suggestions, preparations, or procedures discussed in this book. Should the reader have any questions concerning the appropriateness of any procedure or preparation mentioned, the author and publisher strongly suggest consulting a professional health care advisor.

Library of Congress Cataloging-in-Publication Data

Crawford, Amanda McQuade.
    The herbal menopause book : herbs, nutrition, and other natural therapies /
by Amanda McQuade Crawford.
        p. cm.
    Includes index.
    ISBN 0-89594-799-4 (pbk.)
    1. Menopause—Alternative treatment.   2. Herbs—Therapeutic use.
3. Naturopathy.   I. Title.
    RG186.C73   1996   96-23416
    618.1'7506—dc20   CIP

Contents

INTRODUCTION

Though excellent books on menopause are available, many giving herbal recommendations, no one book covers all the questions and concerns of the millions of women in the West who are embarking on, experiencing, or moving past this major life transition. *The Herbal Menopause Book* focuses on herbs, nutrition, and other natural approaches for perimenopause—the time leading up to and including the Change—and the postmenopausal years. With this book, I hope to increase women's knowledge about the choices they have in natural therapies for menopausal conditions. This book is for women following conventional therapies who may come away with an expanded view of their health-care options. It is also for women already well versed in the simplicity and efficacy of herbal medicine. For all women and their health-care providers who are unsure but interested in using herbs during menopause, this book suggests different answers to age-old questions: What can herbal therapy do for menopause? Can it replace conventional Western medical therapy? Can the two be used together? These are the most commonly asked questions when women are first considering natural remedies. The answers are all encouraging.

Herbal therapy, in contrast to conventional hormone replacement therapy (HRT), offers safer self-care for common symptoms, along with the added confidence a woman feels from being in control of how strong she makes her herbal medicine. In a very real way, herbs joyfully offer a woman the support of all nature and all her predecessors during her natural Change. Herbs, wise nutrition choices, and other therapies that have recently been termed "holistic" have in fact been practiced by women around the world since the Stone Age. We do not yet have documented studies of all our best healing plants and foods, but we have thousands of woman-years of use from which to learn. The more recent use of either equine hormones (natural hormones from horses) or synthetic hormones in conventional medical practice assumes that menopause is a deficiency of estrogen caused by a failure of the ovaries. In fact, we are following our bodies' design for self-preservation when the ovaries decrease circulating levels of estrogen at this time of life. Herbs can work in concert with allopathic medicine or, over time, perhaps even replace it entirely. The strongest argument in favor of herbal therapy is that, contrary to conventional medicine, menopause is not considered a disease to be treated, but a natural stage in the evolution of every woman's life—to be celebrated, not medicated.

This book devotes a chapter to each of four main areas of concern: premenopause, menopause, hormone replacement therapy and its related concerns, and postmenopause. Each chapter includes general discussions of conditions and their causes followed by effective natural health-care recommendations: herbal combinations, nutritional advice, and other helpful information and techniques.

Chapter 1, "Premenopause," describes the physical changes as a woman enters the menopausal period: hormonal changes, decline of fertility, erratic menstrual cycles, spotting and flooding, fibroids, and changes in sexuality. The chapter also discusses mood swings and other ways in which erratic hormone levels affect our emotions, our physical health, and all of who we are.

Chapter 2, "Menopause," describes the conditions most commonly experienced by women at menopause. It provides advice on preventing heart disease and osteoporosis, and then addresses the discomforts women may experience during this period: depression, difficult and painful menstrual cycles (including menstrual migraines and headaches), hot flashes, and night sweats. The remedies and recommendations in the chapter are specific to menopause itself but may be used throughout the perimenopausal period. Because the menstrual cycle undergoes major changes after premenopause, the chapter suggests additional herbal support to rebalance women's changing rhythms. Finally, there are brief sections on herbal remedies to help with the changing appearance of skin and hair and with vaginal thinning and dryness.

Chapter 3, "Hormone Replacement Therapy," reviews the advantages, disadvantages, and history of HRT to help women decide if it is right for them. This chapter also discusses "hormones from herbs," natural hormone replacement, and premature menopause caused by illness or, more commonly, by surgical removal of the ovaries (as in a total hysterectomy). At the end of this chapter is a section for women who choose to come off HRT with the use of herbs. This can be done safely, but I've listed reasons both for and against it, as well as the herbs to be used should this be the course decided upon. The more information a woman has at her disposal, the better able she'll be to provide herself with safe self-healing.

Chapter 4, "Postmenopause," focuses on the concerns of women during the many years after their last menstrual cycle. The most common health need during this stage of life is for natural ways to manage arthritis and joint pain. Because older women also have changing nutritional needs, the chapter offers herbal remedies for bloating, indigestion, and weight gain. Memory loss or unclear thinking is another major concern for which nourishing, toning herbs are ideally suited. The older woman who experiences occasional insomnia and may or may not be taking other medications will find safe and effective recommendations here. Immune strength begins with general resistance, so the chapter also suggests ways to build resistance to avoid colds and flus, bladder infections, and shingles, an infection to which older women are prone, as well as remedies to use when these conditions occur. Finally, Chapter 4 includes optional ways to nourish the complexion and minimize vaginal thinning or dryness. Though this chapter does not cover every immune or health event that the mature woman may face, it does address those conditions I see most often in my practice.

Following these chapters is the "Materia Medica," a layperson's dictionary of the herbs found in this book. Each major herb used in a formula for internal use in this book is listed here alphabetically by its common name, followed by alternate common names and the herb's botanical, or Latin, name. Each entry contains information about the parts of the plant that are used in herbal preparations, conditions the herb is good for and why, recommended doses of teas and tinctures, and any cautions that a reader should know. No toxic herbs are included in this book; some of the stronger herbs are quite safe for women to use at home as recommended in the specific formulas and the "Materia Medica." A few herbs mentioned in passing are not found in the "Materia Medica," but are simply described in the text where they appear.

Appendix A provides guidelines for preparing herbs: how to brew a perfect pot of therapeutic herb tea, how to make extracts, herbal oils, and all the other herbal preparations described in this book. For the adventurous woman or one who already uses herbs, Appendix B explains how to make your own herbal menopause formula, just in case those in this book don't suit all your needs. Appendix C suggests herbs for your home medicine chest. The resources section lists herb suppliers, organizations, educational sources, and publications that you may want to investigate. The bibliography includes publications I relied upon in writing this book, as well as those that may be of further interest to you.

How to Use This Book

Each explanation of a symptom, imbalance, or health challenge presented in this book is followed by an "Herbal Medicine" that in most cases provides two herbal medicine formulas. These are usually very similar to each other: one is a tea (for those women seeking an alcohol-free option) and the other uses the same or almost the same herbs, only in the form of a concentrated extract.

The first recipe given for each condition is designed to be formulated from store-bought, alcohol-based extracts, which require the least fuss and act most quickly, but are more expensive than teas. If, for example, you need help with debilitating hot flashes or brutal mood swings, take the tincture formula from this book to your nearest herb shop and buy the extracts off the shelf. Tinctures are also more convenient than brewing up a pot of less-expensive herb tea on a consistent basis.

The second herbal formula, a tea, is more effective and affordable over time, though it may not work fast enough for the headache or hot flash requiring immediate attention. Milder because they are extracted in hot water instead of alcohol, each gentle dose of tea adds up, over time, to more long-lasting health. Also, the extra water that tea provides allows your body more freedom to take up what it needs and excrete what is not needed. Water-soluble herbal constituents are the mildest way to care for yourself. If you are sensitive to medications, you may prefer to start with teas.

If your symptoms come and go, you can, if you like, take both tea and extracts at the same time; there is no risk of overdose if you follow the guidelines given in this book.

Note: Whether you have one menopausal symptom or twenty, choose the herbal formula that focuses on your worst symptom first. After years of clinical herbal practice helping women through the Change, I have found that, as a general rule, one formula addressing your worst symptom first will extend to relieve accompanying imbalances.

After the "Herbal Medicine" section for each health challenge, you'll find a "Nutrition" section that offers suggestions for whole foods that provide vitamins and minerals to address each particular health imbalance. If these problems respond well to natural supplements, the appropriate supplements are listed as well. This is the most conservative aspect of the holistic treatment plan presented in this book because, in my opinion, less is often more when it comes to taking manufactured products. There are other books encouraging more dependence on megadoses of supernutrients, but I prefer to emphasize whole foods and can include only what my experience leads me to recommend. If readers are surprised by my omission of standard supplements, I beg your pardon. I view supplements as just that—supplements to wise nutrition choices and safely monitored botanical balancing.

Finally, the "In Addition" section for each health issue provides further helpful natural therapies. Guided imagery and visualization have helped many women in my practice, and I have included several to try in "In Addition" sections throughout this book. Also included are recipes for therapeutic external creams, salves, and herbal oils; specific exercises; and hints for making positive changes in your daily life.

In closing, let me say that, while the recommendations in this book are based on my experience as a medical herbalist, please know that I am not at odds with modern Western medicine. I work with all types of healers—medical doctors, acupuncturists, midwives, nurse practitioners, naturopaths, and other herbalists. My abiding belief is that health care is really about the choices we make—not just what health plan or type of practitioner we choose, but the way we choose to live our lives outside the doctor's office. To me, taking the time to sit under a tree can be as important as the drugs you choose to take (or herbs, for that matter). If adhering to an allopathic course of treatment for menopause makes you feel safe, I will not be the one to say you have chosen unwisely. On the contrary, my experience with women of all ages has shown me that, given the room, the chance, and the power to make their own informed, well-thought-out decisions, women usually choose the right path for themselves. It is my duty to help them along that path, which may mean suggesting a gentle tea for night sweats or a strong herbal regimen to help wean them off HRT. Herbalism is not in conflict or competition with standard medicine, at least not the type of herbalism I practice. Closed-mindedness is our only true enemy. So please, feel free to show your health professional this book, but be prepared for a less-than-enthusiastic response from most doctors. If they can't support you in making your own informed decision, may I suggest you get a second opinion.

Finally, this book is not meant for the coffee table. It is a self-help manual, which means it is to be used. If it gets stained with spilled tea or dog-eared by many hands, then I will consider the whole undertaking to have been worthwhile.

Chapter 1

PREMENOPAUSE

Menopause occurs when the ovaries stop releasing eggs and menstruation ceases. The period called "premenopause" can begin eight to ten years before complete menopause and occurs when the normal monthly cycle of ovulation and menstruation becomes less regular. This entire period of transition is also known as the *climacteric* because the reproductive phase of life is reaching its "climax." The formal term is *perimenopause*—which means, literally, the time surrounding menopausal changes.

The changes that accompany menopause are no less dramatic than those you experienced at puberty. Your body is changing, and along with those changes come new, strange feelings. All these changes are perfectly natural and normal, and they are occurring throughout your body. To help you understand the menopausal change, the first part of this chapter discusses what is happening to your body at the cellular level. To help you adapt to your changing body, the second part of the chapter provides practical, effective guidance that you can apply during the premenopausal period and throughout this new stage of life.

The Reproductive Process and Premenopause

Our reproductive systems undergo natural, predictable changes from puberty to menopause. Each month after puberty and until menopause, a woman's ovaries normally produce one egg, and the lining of the uterus thickens to prepare for a developing fetus if conception occurs. If conception does not occur, this uterine lining (endometrium) is discarded and released as menstrual blood.

Our endocrine systems produce hormones that circulate in our bodies and stimulate different functional activities at the cellular level. Estrogen, the hormone produced by a developing egg, is key to the functions and changes in a woman's reproductive system. Women enter puberty when the body begins to produce significant levels of estrogen, and enter menopause when the body gradually stops producing as much.

When we are still having menstrual cycles, we are low in estrogen just before bleeding, especially on the first day. This is true whether you are twenty-two or forty-two. The brain senses low levels of estrogen in the blood and sends a message to the pituitary gland in the brain to release "follicle-stimulating hormone" (FSH) into the bloodstream. FSH runs on down to visit the ovaries and stimulates development of an egg within its surrounding cavity (follicle). As the egg develops, it makes estrogen, so levels in the bloodstream start to rise. This signals the brain that it can stop firing such a strong message to the pituitary.

Meanwhile, back in the ovary, the developing egg keeps maturing while several others die off and turn into surrounding ovarian tissue. The FSH decreases as the egg's secretion of estrogen signals the brain not to send so much FSH, but the FSH that is still being sent to the ovaries keeps the one egg growing, which ensures that the level of estrogen keeps rising for now. The egg creates enough estrogen by about Day 14 to trigger a release of "luteinizing hormone" (LH) from the pituitary. LH causes more blood to circulate into the ovaries, bringing about two important changes. One, more cholesterol (a normal sterol found in the blood) is broken down in the ovaries and eventually changed into even more estrogen. Two, enzymes help liberate the fully mature egg from its follicle for ovulation. The empty follicle now folds in on itself to form a soft lump, called the *corpus luteum*, "yellow body"—yellow because of its fatty sterols, which are now made into a different female sex hormone, progesterone, the pro-gestation hormone that acts to prepare the uterus for implantation of the egg, to maintain pregnancy, and to promote milk production in the breasts.

If there is no fertilization of the egg (now waiting around in the fallopian tubes for a date), the corpus luteum learns this through the chemistry of the blood. In turn, the corpus luteum stops making progesterone.

In premenopause, there are fewer viable eggs than in past years and the ovaries become less responsive to FSH and LH. Some cycles never have enough estrogen built up for ovulation, although menstrual bleeding may still occur. Our bodies begin to need much less estrogen than was required for menstruation, conception, pregnancy, and lactation. But we do not completely lose all estrogen in menopause. A healthy cushion of body fat provides some estrogen, and the adrenal glands also make a little. A lower level of estrogen may even have important advantages. As cycles become more irregular, estrogen-dependent symptoms such as painful cramps, tender breasts, menstrual migraines, and heavy bleeding from fibroids tend to improve. On the other hand, symptoms of low estrogen may potentially create new problems—at least until our bodies reach a new balance. Since estrogen is only one of many hormones whose levels are changing, herbs that promote progesterone have also helped "low estrogen" symptoms of menopause, presumably by supporting our bodies in reaching that new balance.

The Onset of Premenopause

Premenopause is usually a gradual process, so women may not know exactly when it begins. If you are reasonably healthy and are older than thirty-six, your irregular cycle may be a sign of premenopause.

Premenopause commonly begins in the forties but may start as early as the thirties or even the twenties. High-stress lifestyles, heightened economic and social worries, global pollution, rising gynecological surgeries, and other late-twentieth-century stresses may contribute to early onset of premenopause, even among healthy women. In addition, the earlier your periods began (called "menarche"), the earlier menopause may occur.

You can determine your probable age at premenopause and the difficulty or ease you will experience by talking to other women in your family. This can be invaluable information. Other factors to consider are personal health history, nutrition, ethnicity, climate, economic status, and social setting, all of which influence one another. For example, women who smoke or make a habit of eating fast food are more likely to have some degree of nutrient imbalance when the Change arrives, and therefore more severe symptoms such as hot flashes, a drop in energy, and dry skin. A history of health problems is associated with an earlier menopause. Keep in mind also that health factors other than premenopause can also make the menstrual cycle erratic—for example, traveling, illness, malnourishment, or rigorous athletic training.

A New Stage of Life

For many women, premenopause is a time of emotional ups and downs. Entering a new stage of life as well as coping with changing hormonal levels naturally make this a time for reevaluating life goals—assessing past accomplishments and defining or redefining the future.

You may wonder why, when you have been perfectly content with your beliefs up until now, you are suddenly questioning everything about your purpose in life and the way you have chosen to conduct it. And you feel quite alone in your observations: You may feel you are the only one to notice that the weather is all wrong, that your favorite dish doesn't taste quite right. You catch your loved ones looking at you funny, which naturally makes you want to send them to summer camp though they are far too old for that now. Meanwhile, you are worrying about aging, and on top of that, you have other challenges to face: family difficulties that tax your resources, career and financial choices to be assessed. When Tuesday's "I'm proud I did the best I could" clashes with Friday's "I've been on the planet for almost half a century and what have I got to show for it?" stop and take a deep breath. These and a myriad of variations on having the emotional rug pulled out from under you are not necessarily signs of disease. Your distress could well be the opening stanza of premenopause.

You should keep in mind that there is no healthy way to suppress your strong emotions during this period. The best you can do is take a mental health holiday, even for five or ten minutes during a hectic schedule. Recognize your need for time to cool off, reflect, and get some space—and then find a way to do it. By tuning in to what you are feeling, you will probably come to identify the known and unknown triggers that bring out these strange feelings and delve beneath the surface of your deeper unease. If you can take the time to muse on things until an insight rings true, you may even come to see the wisdom in this seeming madness. The process may be helped along with a relaxing herb tea, a counseling session, or ten minutes locked in a bathroom stall breathing slowly and evenly. Premenopause does not make women "crazy," it makes us look inside. If we don't look inside, we will soon *feel crazy*.

At any stage of premenopause, gentle herbal self-care can help realign your essential, unchanging self with your emerging physical, emotional, mental, and spiritual changes. Less ideally, you can use megadoses of herbal supplements as natural drugs to "fix" a premenopausal symptom, whether it is a mood change or an irregular cycle. The herbal drug approach can work for some women. But if we embrace the rite of passage that menopause represents and take advantage of this special opportunity for deep transformation, we really should not suppress the symptoms. Drugs, natural or pharmaceutical, are fine for short-term fixes, but, as you might guess, have hidden costs, such as side effects needing still more treatment. Many of these are discussed in Chapter 3, "Hormone Replacement Therapy."

The rest of this chapter explores some of the most common challenges faced during premenopause. Some are symptoms that alarm women; some are more general signs of physical change you can observe in yourself; and some are nonphysical results of body changes that manifest as emotional or mental self-doubts. Many more changes than these may occur while a woman is wondering whether she has entered menopause. Hot flashes, weight gain, and episodes of depression may occur in either premenopause or menopause; these are covered in Chapter 2, "Menopause."

Mood Swings

When women speak of mood swings, they often mean depression, anxiety, or irritability, not upward swings of elation or joy. But you can experience both extremes under the biochemical influence of fluctuating hormones. If you want to fully experience your changing feelings without suppressing them or being run ragged by your emotions when they surface, try the following nonaggressive herbal remedies. The key to their effectiveness is consistency: Over time, these gentle herbal allies can help restore balance to your nervous system and hormonal cycle.

Whether this gentle approach works depends on four factors: how long your stress level has driven your mood swings up and down, how troubling these emotional changes feel to you, how quickly or slowly your unique chemistry responds to the herbs, and what other steps you take to complement the healing herbs. As soon as all symptoms feel better or are almost gone (usually after two to three months), continue the same combination and dose for an extra three weeks; then reduce the dose by half for another three weeks. If you feel just as well after reducing the amount this way, simply keep a little extra on hand for future times when an occasional week back on the herbs will help you cope with a rough spell. If you should have any lingering symptoms after four or five months, continue taking the herbs at half dose five days a week. When you feel ready, try reducing the dose again. Watch how well you respond, and skip the tea when your moods feel stable to you.

Herbal Medicine

❦ ───── MOTHER THE LIONHEARTED ───── ❦

Extracts	Botanical Names	Actions
2 oz. motherwort herb	*Leonurus cardiaca*	Calms heart palpitations; cooling
2 oz. skullcap herb	*Scutellaria laterifolia*	Reduces anxiety, tension headaches
2 oz. Siberian ginseng root	*Eleutherococcus senticosus*	Increases natural resistance to stress
2 oz. St. John's wort herb	*Hypericum perforatum*	Lifts depression; repairs frayed nerves
2 oz. black cohosh root	*Cimicifuga racemosa*	Calms nerves; helps balance hormones

Ten ounces will last thirty days. Combine these herbal extracts. Take 1 teaspoon in 1 cup water in the morning and evening. Take an additional dropperful every ten minutes as needed during stressful days or for better sleep at night. For chronic stress, take for a minimum of two months before expecting lasting benefits. For best effect, take full dosage over six months and then half-strength for another four months.

❦ ───── LOVE MY LIFE TEA ───── ❦

Dried Herbs	Botanical Names	Actions
5 oz. skullcap herb	*Scutellaria laterifolia*	Reduces anxiety, tension headaches
5 oz. lemon balm leaf	*Melissa officinalis*	Lifts depression; good for immunity, taste
3 oz. passion flower vine	*Passiflora incarnata*	Lessens physical, emotional pain
2 oz. chamomile flower	*Matricaria recutita*	Calms effects of stress on digestion

Fifteen ounces will last thirty days. Add 1/2 ounce to 3 1/2 cups of boiling water in a teapot or container with a well-fitting lid. Let stand for fifteen minutes before straining. Drink 1 cup hot or cold three times a day. If you prefer, sip tea throughout the day or drink two larger glasses twice a day, making sure you drink 3 cups in a day.

Nutrition

Wise Food Choices

- Choose foods high in vitamin C: red, green, yellow bell peppers; fresh broccoli; citrus fruits; rosehip jam (although vitamin C is lost in cooking except in some high-quality brands, natural fruit pectins and bioflavonoids offer other benefits); baked potatoes.
- For healthy nerves, eat foods high in B complex: dark green leafy vegetables and whole grains such as brown rice, polenta, buckwheat, whole wheat with bran, and wheat germ.
- Eat one clove of raw or lightly steamed garlic in food daily to protect the heart from long-term stress. Fresh garlic provides zinc, chromium, and other nutrients, and it kills off microbes. Cooked garlic and deodorized garlic capsules benefit the heart but have fewer immune benefits.
- Reduce animal fats and excess protein. Calcium from dairy foods and iron from meat is not well used when a woman is under chronic stress, so eating more doesn't add energy.
- Replace chicken or red meat with tofu, tempeh, or other soy protein one to two times a week.
- Occasionally add 1 teaspoon to 1 tablespoon sesame seeds or tahini (the delicious paste of ground sesame seeds) to salads; use tahini on crackers instead of margarine or butter. For a vegetable dip or satisfying nondairy sandwich spread, mix 1/3 cup tahini into a paste with 1 tablespoon water and 1 to 2 teaspoons miso (rice, barley, or soybean paste) to taste. Sesame seeds are high in calcium and other nutrients, and its oil provides essential fatty acids; though women concerned with weight gain and heart health are well advised to lower dietary fats, we do require some healthy oils for good nerve function and immunity. When we feel nourished and eat small amounts of these concentrated, healthy plant oils, our craving for inappropriate fats lessens. For those who are interested, the use of sesame seed has ancient spiritual reverberations associated with physical protection.

Supplements

- Vitamin A, beta-carotene; dose depends on individual woman
- Vitamin B complex
- Vitamin C
- Folic acid
- Balanced calcium and magnesium (see "Osteoporosis" in Chapter 2, "Menopause")

- Deodorized garlic capsules as directed on labels if you prefer them to steamed or raw garlic in food

In Addition

- Occasionally work in the garden for half an hour (but if you enjoy gardening, you know that a half hour can stretch into hours because getting your hands in the dirt is so relaxing and weeding gets out so much tension).
- Especially if you don't have a garden, stretch for ten minutes on the floor before crawling into bed.
- Take four drops of Tiger Lily flower essence (available from the Flower Essence Society; see "Resources") four times a day, or use it in your bathwater for added relaxation.
- Make a huge, double-strength batch of hot chamomile tea (4 to 8 ounces of herb in 1 to 2 quarts of water); strain and reserve 1 cup for sipping, adding a little honey if you wish. Pour the rest into a hot bath. Light a candle, turn off the lights, and relax for at least fifteen minutes. Alternatively, mix 4 to 8 drops of chamomile or lavender essential oil into a tub of water and soak away the tension of the day.
- Only have a shower? Put 3 drops of any essential oil on a wash cloth; holding it under the stream of water about 10 inches from your face, gently breathe in the steam. Then wash your body with this lightly scented cloth instead of soap.

Erratic Menstrual Cycles

As you enter premenopause, you may experience erratic menstrual cycles. Menstrual bleeding continues as long as the ovaries secrete some estrogen because the hormone builds up the uterine lining (endometrium), which later leaves the body as menstrual blood. Meanwhile, your body is adjusting to its new hormonal balance in the following way. Most of the eggs your ovaries contained at birth have been used one way or another by now for pregnancies or nonpregnant menstrual flows. Some have naturally died off with every ovulation. A few viable eggs may still be present at this point, but ovulation is erratic. If an egg is not developing, there is no ovulation. Without ovulation, there is a drop in progesterone, which is even more significant than the drop in estrogen. For a while during premenopause it can be normal to have a higher level of both FSH and LH in the blood, but without enough progesterone, the pituitary gland in the brain sends out less and less LH. Why? Perhaps the pituitary knows better than to keep on trying to stimulate an egg to develop in a follicle if it senses biochemically that the egg is not there. The lack of this ovarian hormone is what informs "headquarters" in the pituitary. Just to be sure, the FSH from the brain takes up the slack by increasing its level in the bloodstream, to get at least some response, if possible, out of the ovaries. In good time, FSH production runs out, too. This is perhaps why herbs that seem to promote progesterone are as important for postponing menopause as herbs that seem to promote estrogen. Fortunately, these herbs are not as strong as pharmaceutical replacement hormones, so they tend to promote only those levels of hormones that the body is capable of utilizing in a healthy way.

Herbs with progestational or estrogenic effects often balance erratic timing of the cycle. With their assistance, irregularities need not be so extreme or occur so suddenly that they embarrass a woman who thought she was "all done" with menstruation. Nor does the transition have to be so irregular that it causes panic in the dignified matron who worries that she may have conceived. But herbs cannot work against nature. No vegetable matter on this planet can put an egg back in an ovary for fertilization. Nor can any healing plant force the uterine lining to build up and flow out again after a woman is past her time for menstruation. On the other hand, there are many documented cases of women who have not bled for a year or longer and then taken hormonally active herbs only to have their menstrual flow resume. Sometimes this was desirable and sometimes not. Rather than overstimulating the uterus, the herbs may have been acting as subtle biological nutrition for a woman with some remaining egg follicles and borderline hormone levels. In this case the hormonal herbs simply allow the uterine lining that has built up over time without monthly release to be cleared out in a few unscheduled menstrual flows.

If you are new to the world of herbs, you should know that there is no reason to be afraid of the following herb teas. They will not cause dangerous postmenopausal bleeding. Medicinal plants are powerful, but unlike poisonous plants or pharmaceutical drugs, these herbs are subject to the body's own healthy self-regulation.

Herbal Medicine

❦————————ANCIENT CLOCK, PERFECT TIMING————————❦

Extracts	Botanical Names	Actions
4 oz. chasteberry seed	*Vitex agnus-castus*	Promotes pituitary control over timing of cycle
3 oz. lady's mantle herb	*Alchemilla vulgaris*	Relaxing reproductive tonic
2 oz. blue cohosh root	*Caulophyllum thalictroides*	Stimulates regular menses
1 oz. nettle leaf	*Urtica dioica*	Provides minerals, nutrition to all cells

Ten ounces will last thirty days. Combine these herbal extracts. Take 1 teaspoon in 1 cup water in the morning and evening.

Dried Herbs	Botanical Names	Actions
4 oz. chasteberry seed	*Vitex agnus-castus*	Promotes pituitary control over timing of cycle
3 oz. lady's mantle herb	*Alchemilla vulgaris*	Relaxing reproductive tonic
2 oz. blue cohosh root	*Caulophyllum thalictroides*	Stimulates regular menses
3 oz. nettle leaf	*Urtica dioica*	Provides minerals, nutrition to all cells
3 oz. rosemary leaf	*Rosmarinus officinalis*	Aids digestion; for flavor

Fifteen ounces will last thirty days. Add 1/2 ounce of the mixture to 3 1/2 cups of boiling water in a teapot or container with a well-fitting lid. Let stand for fifteen minutes before straining. Drink 1 cup hot or cold three times a day. If you prefer, sip tea throughout the day or drink two larger glasses twice a day, but be sure to drink 3 cups in a day.

Nutrition

Wise Food Choices

- Avoid fats, especially heated oils and animal fats such as those in cheese and red meat.
- Avoid excess protein, packaged convenience foods, refined flour, sugar, and junk food.
- Eat three carrots or drink 10 ounces fresh carrot juice daily for a week before you expect to bleed, even if that part of the monthly cycle is early or late.
- Eat sweet potatoes, yams, or baked organic potatoes (your choice) three times a week.
- Add 1/2 to 1 teaspoon or even just a sprinkling of fennel seeds to Italian or East Indian sauces and dishes, such as rice pilaf and polenta with sun-dried tomatoes.
- Eat salads with cucumber, chopped onion, dill, and lemon juice, to taste.

Supplements

- Evening primrose oil. Because capsules may vary in milligrams, the dose is actually a range. A minimum dose, 6 to 10 capsules of 500 milligrams or more each a day, is expensive, but this supplement may be needed only for six weeks or so, making it more practical and affordable. While some reports suggest that even 2 to 4 capsules a day help some women, most experienced care providers agree that fewer than 8 or 10 capsules per day is a waste of money, so economizing in this way may not be a gain. Also, borage and black currant oil are cheaper sources of GLA (gamma linoleic acid), but effects vary; so follow recommended dosages on labels.

- Home-sprouted seeds and legumes of every kind cost only pennies a day and are a great alternative to evening primrose oil. Sprouted seeds and raw nuts provide easily digested plant protein and good-quality essential fatty acids in a water-based form we can handle, in addition to enzymes helpful to good metabolism.

In Addition

- Try the "Ten-Minute Visualization" (see box below).

Ten-Minute Visualization

Don't just read this—try it, trusting in your body's ancient wisdom to benefit from this and every effort you make to bring healing from within. Perhaps you could make a tape of yourself speaking the following words and listen to them every day. If you record the visualization, you may wish to leave a silent pause of thirty seconds or more where asterisks (*) appear. Routinely practicing this visualization allows your whole spirit, mind, and body to reset your biological clock gently but firmly over a twenty-eight-day lunar cycle. You may also use this visualization whenever you need to get centered.

Breathe deeply, exhaling all your thoughts and worries. Breathe in. Let it all go while you straighten your spine. On your next in-breath, count to three. * Count to three as you breathe out. * Repeat this for the next few minutes, for a total of 21 times. * Count to four as you breathe in. * Count to four as you breathe out. * Repeat this once. * Allow your breath to continue evenly and slowly, in and out. In and out. You are sitting in perfect balance in a comfortable darkness. Continue to breathe evenly and slowly. *

With every in-breath, the darkness fades up to a deep and lovely blue. With every out-breath, the sky fills slowly with light, until you can see the whole Earth from where you sit. Breathe in and out. * Watch your breathing seem to draw the sun as it appears over the horizon. Breathe it down into the sea at sunset. Breathe in and out seven times in stillness and peace.

With your next in-breath, see the moon rise over the Earth's horizon. Breathe in evenly, breathe out slowly so the moon can glide up effortlessly. * When the moon is at its highest so the moonbeams splash down on you, it will start to set. When its silver-violet light has entirely disappeared, breathe in and out in comfortable darkness seven times. Then you will know it is time to gently open your eyes. *

There is something about this "timeout" that seems to create a sense of having more time. Each time you follow this exercise for aligning with your natural timing, you will be using your own creative impulse to gain in health and inner peace.

Spotting and Flooding

During premenopause, you may notice that the time between periods is shorter, but the flow is less than in the past. These spotty periods may alternate with normal cycles or be replaced by sudden, gushing bleeding (flooding) for five to eight days. In itself, heavy blood loss isn't abnormal, but it is wise to have a trusted health-care provider rule out other causes, such as fibroids or malignancy. Three or four extremely heavy flows in a row can cause anemia. Even if anemia is only temporary, you can follow the recommendations below to correct or prevent it. If you lose a lot more blood than you normally do each month, pay attention to other signs of anemia, such as a pale tongue and inner edges of eyelids, fatigue, cold hands and feet, shallow breathing, or minor cuts and wounds that take a long time to heal.

Herbal Medicine

❧————————————TAMING SEVEN SEAS FORMULA————————————❧

Extracts	Botanical Names	Actions
4 oz. shepherd's purse herb	*Capsella bursapastoris*	Fresh plant best anti-hemorrhagic
3 oz. lady's mantle herb	*Alchemilla vulgaris*	Astringent; calming; uterine tonic
2 oz. yellow dock root	*Rumex crispus*	Promotes liver function; adds iron
1 oz. blue cohosh root	*Caulophyllum thalictroides*	Stops spasms; balances hormonal signals

Ten ounces will last thirty days. Combine these herbal extracts. Take 1 teaspoon in 1 cup water in the morning and evening. Take an extra dropperful every ten minutes until excess bleeding slows or stops.

❧———————————— OCEAN WAVE, CALM TIDES————————————❧

Dried Herbs	Botanical Names	Actions
3 oz. lady's mantle herb	*Alchemilla vulgaris*	Tones bleeding uterine walls; balances and calms
3 oz. raspberry leaf	*Rubus idaeus*	Slows blood loss; replaces lost fluid and calcium
3 oz. nettle leaf	*Urtica dioica*	Replaces lost fluids; rich in minerals, vitamins
4 oz. rosehips	*Rosa canina*	Vitamin C for iron, mineral assimilation; for taste
1/2 oz. rose flowers	*Rosa species*	Organically grown buds or petals reduce bleeding, infection
1 1/2 oz. sage leaf	*Salvia officinalis*	Hormone balancing; astringent; aids digestion

Fifteen ounces will last thirty days. Add 1/2 ounce of the mixture to 3 1/2 cups boiling water in a teapot or container with a well-fitting lid. Let stand for fifteen minutes before straining. Drink 1 cup hot or cold three times a day. You may sip tea throughout the day or drink two larger glasses twice a day, but be sure you drink 3 cups a day.

Nutrition

Wise Food Choices

Occasional heavy blood loss or prolonged spotting can lead to anemia. To prevent it, obtain iron from food sources, which won't cause constipation as supplements often do:

- Unsulphured apricots soaked for fifteen minutes or longer in water
- Ten raw pumpkin seeds a day on salads or as a quick-energy snack
- Blackstrap molasses, 1 tablespoon drizzled over old-fashioned (not microwaved or instant) oatmeal on cold mornings
- One-eighth teaspoon cinnamon on applesauce on warm mornings or for late-night snacks instead of sweets or bread
- A dash of red cayenne pepper to taste whenever practical in salad dressing, on grains or soups

  Alternatively, for short-term effects against spotting and bleeding, mix 1/4 teaspoon cayenne powder in 2 teaspoons honey; knock back quickly, with a chaser of water, tomato juice, or some other juice you like, four times a day for one to three days or until flooding stops. This remedy will not burn the stomach even though it may feel like it initially. To avoid the use of honey, take 1/4 teaspoon cayenne powder wrapped in edible starch papers, available at natural-food stores, or take the pepper in capsules (less reliable), 6 "00" size, four times a day with water, juice, or a piece of plain bread to assist digestion. If you do not see any benefits in a few hours to one day, check with your health-care provider.
- Red, yellow, and green vegetables, especially steamed kale and spinach
- Root vegetables: burdock chopped like carrots in soup, grated beets or jicama in salads
- Nasturtium flowers and leaves, watercress added to salads

In Addition

- Rest frequently during spotting or flooding. Raise the legs and feet on a few pillows above the head and heart.
- Every night for a week take a bath (not too hot) containing 5 drops each of these essential oils: chamomile, lavender, clary sage. Do this even if you have only one or two oils.

- Sell your television and watch clouds instead (better plots).
- Excuse yourself from work for an hour or two ("Something has come up") or leave a friendly but clear message on your phone indicating that you are in conference or otherwise occupied and unavailable. Then go talk with your guardian angels for an hour. After that you can catch up on any urgent tasks or pleasant projects with mind and body renewed.

Decline of Fertility

You may find yourself entering premenopause and experiencing a reduction in fertility but still wanting to have a child. Although there is a popular belief that having a baby later in life entails unacceptable health risks, there is no real reason to assume that a healthy forty-year-old, for example, is "lucky" to experience a normal pregnancy. In fact, a woman experiencing premenopause in her thirties and early forties will most likely have a safe pregnancy. Recent studies indicate that the increase in Downs syndrome babies born to women over forty, though established, is not necessarily due to the age of the ovum. At age forty, chances are 1 in 100 that a mother will give birth to a Downs child, but, conversely, that also means the child will be normal 99 times out of 100. Other theories suggest that the age of male partners, frequency of intercourse, and external cofactors such as X-rays, environmental toxins, and illness may play a role in the incidence of Downs.

Today, plenty of noninvasive support is available to women who face declining fertility but want to have a child. Women wise in the ways of herbal medicine have known for millennia which plants are best for restoring natural functions. A first blessing on your intention to conceive is to take the following combination of herbal extracts. A second blessing comes with each simple cup of womb-honoring herbal tea. During menstruation, skip the extract but continue with the herbal tea. If conception occurs, continue with the tea only.

In general, use the following combinations for a minimum of three months. You can safely take these herbs for up to five years, although most women will need them for only one to two years. If you take them for more than two years, skip the regimen one day a week to give your metabolism a rest.

If you feel a deep need to be important in the life of a child and natural pregnancy is not possible, by all means work to find alternative ways to "mother." Many, many women consider life without children to provide other riches; some women teach their own special skills to children in community groups; others adopt or offer loving homes as foster parents to children who desperately need them. Seek and you will find your own special way.

Herbal Medicine

RECIPE FOR AN ANGEL

Extracts	Botanical Names	Actions
3 oz. chasteberry seed	*Vitex agnus-castus*	Promotes conception
2 oz. dong quai root	*Angelica sinensis*	Balances estrogen; warms, nourishes circulation
4 oz. raspberry leaf	*Rubus idaeus*	Nourishing uterine tonic; calcium rich, calming
1 oz. black cohosh	*Cimicifuga racemosa*	Eases muscle spasms and mental or physical tension

Combine these herbal extracts. Take 1 teaspoon in 1 cup water twice per day, in the morning and evening; 10 ounces will last approximately thirty days.

ROOT-TO-FRUIT BREW

Dried Herbs	Botanical Names	Actions
4 oz. sarsaparilla root	*Smilax ornata*	Balances hormones; cleanses skin; supports lymph, immunity
4 oz. raspberry leaf	*Rubus idaeus*	Nourishing tonic; provides calcium
3 oz. red clover flower	*Trifolium pratense*	Promotes estrogenic balance and fertility
4 oz. rosehips	*Rosa canina*	Bioflavonoids promote tissue repair

Add 1/2 ounce of the mixture to 3 1/2 cups of boiling water in a teapot or other container with a tight-fitting lid. Let stand for fifteen minutes before straining. Drink 1 cup hot or cold three times per day; 15 ounces will last approximately thirty days. If you prefer, sip the tea throughout the day, or drink two larger glasses in the course of a day, but be sure you drink 3 cups total.

Nutrition

Wise Food Choices

- Watermelon, pomegranates, fresh figs, and other fruit with seeds, all in season
- Zucchini, squash, or other vegetables, in soup or stir-fried
- Live green sprouts, such as alfalfa, sunflower, aduki, lentil, fenugreek, and onion

- "Wild weed" salads: dandelion, mustard greens, nettle shoots, lamb's quarters, miner's lettuce, wild lettuce, edible Chinese chrysanthemums
- Homemade nondairy pesto with basil, thyme, olive oil, powdered dulse or kelp, and fresh nuts
- One freshly cracked walnut per day
- One to 3 teaspoons coarsely chopped raw seeds or nuts on salads three times per week
- Soybeans, other soy foods (such as tofu or tempeh), or 1 tablespoon of soy flour mixed with other flours, two to five times per week
- Curried *dahl* with garlic, cumin, turmeric, mild or hot to taste
- For nonvegans and nonvegetarians, two eggs, or 4 ounces lean white fish, or 3 ounces cooked lamb, once a week

   Even though our bodies are quite capable of thriving on a vegetarian diet, there is no getting around the fact that the sterols provided by meat consumption are stimulating to the human endocrine system. Organic animal fats and proteins in moderation can help weak, stressed, or underweight women. (Unfortunately, commercial hormones added to butter, eggs, meat, and cheese make many women feel worse.) To replace this animal energy, vegetarians and vegans need to emphasize the more concentrated plant protein foods suggested in the other categories above.
- Avoid any foods that trigger allergies.

Supplements
- Folic acid
- Vitamin D from natural sunlight (about twenty minutes per day)

   Natural vitamin D synthesis in your body occurs when sunshine is allowed to fall on your skin. This does not mean tanning salons or risking skin cancer at the beach. Taking a walk is an excellent way to supplement vitamin D as well as give yourself some pleasant exercise, which prevents osteoporosis and reduces stress or tension in the body.

In Addition
- To 1 ounce sweet almond oil, add 21 drops essential oil of jasmine. Massage the abdomen, breasts, underarms. For the full treatment worthy of any goddess, occasionally spend one to two hours massaging and soothing tired skin, paying special attention to sore spots as well as stretching and kneading the muscles in the calves, thighs, forearms, and fingers. Perhaps have someone else rub your back, neck, and shoulders.
- Castor oil packs (see box) placed over the abdomen or lower back once or twice a week can help the body self-repair if old scars are blocking conception. The messiness of these packs is worth the cleanup, especially when you consider the bonus of great pelvic circulation.

- Yoga will open the pelvis, as well as prepare ligaments and muscles, for the possibility of pregnancy.
- Create a secret ceremony, known only to you and your lover, to create a receptive mood, to protect the rich bloom of your passion, and to open both of you to the sacred gift of a child.
- Visualizing healthy change and conception has great power here. Many women who are now mothers of healthy children were told that their sonograms or other tests ruled out any reasonable expectation of conception. This is a good time for women to move beyond "reason" to the miracle. We know that our emotions affect our hormones, and that our hormones affect our fertility. Having lost our conscious connection to the body's ways doesn't mean we have lost our subconscious connection to dream, vision, purpose, or love.

Castor Oil Pack

Castor oil, made from the castor bean plant (*Ricinus communis*, also called Palma Christi in folklore), can be used externally in a hot compress to reduce swelling and overgrowths of fibrous tissue. It is available at herb shops, natural-food stores, and some drugstores as well as from many of the suppliers listed in "Resources."

Heat at least 4 ounces of castor oil in a small saucepan or a double boiler. The oil is the right temperature when a drop on your wrist is hot but not uncomfortably so. To avoid burns and grease fires, take special care not to spill the oil. Pour the oil into the center of a hand towel or large piece of flannel, and fold the fabric over once or twice to hold it. Add more oil as needed to saturate the fabric. Place the warm, oily cloth on the skin over the lower abdomen or lower back. It can also help any bruise, swelling, or growth. Lay a hot-water bottle or another clean, dry towel over towel soaked in castor oil to reduce heat loss. Leave it on your skin for twenty minutes to an hour—as long as it remains warm (the hot-water bottle can be refilled as needed; fresh, heated castor oil may be added). Repeat no more than twice a week for severe conditions—the breakdown of tissue should not proceed faster than the body's ability to safely eliminate what is being stirred up. Increased blood flow from the hot oil pack improves general circulation and elimination.

Adding therapeutically fragrant, spiritually uplifting essential oils (*not* chemical perfumes) is especially helpful when stress or depression about self-image accompany infertility, fibroids, and other reproductive conditions. These are not added to the castor oil while it is heating—the essential (volatile) oils would evaporate—but just before it is poured into the towel. For every 3 or 4 ounces of warm castor oil, add 3 to 4 drops each of one or more of the following pure essential oils (available at herb or natural-food stores, or by mail order): geranium, marjoram, clary sage, ginger. They are expensive, but small amounts last a long time.

Sexuality and Vaginal Changes

You may notice some physical changes as your estrogen levels decline during perimenopause, and all of them are perfectly normal and healthy: The fat cushion in the labia is reabsorbed, the smaller lips (*labia minora*) may eventually disappear, the vaginal canal gets a little smaller, the vaginal wall becomes thinner. The cells of the vaginal walls are also less cornified (less tough, which means more sensitive to both pleasant pressure and potential irritation). The place where the top of the vagina folds in on itself to become the cervix gets a little shallower. The size of the cervix also decreases, and the glands in the mucous membrane surfaces throughout the vaginal canal secrete lubricants less actively.

These effects of decreasing estrogen happen over time and vary in degree from woman to woman. But don't believe for a minute that good sex disappears along with these changes. Many postmenopausal women in their sixties and seventies have reported satisfying sex, good lubrication, low incidences of infection, and an abundant, secret well of desire. For many of us, lubrication must now be stimulated by great loving, not just any old hormonal flush of youth. It may take longer to bring the bucket to the top of the well, but, as they say, the water tastes sweeter since it rises from so deep. That thirst is one you can choose to let grow or ignore if there is no lover worthy of your bed. With no fear of pregnancy to put a crimp in your pleasure, you may know full body ecstasy now, even if you haven't known it before. The following combination nourishes the sex drive when it is used in small doses over time and tones the reproductive tissues to optimize sensuality.

Herbal Medicine

TEMPLE GATES ELIXIR

Extracts	Botanical Names	Actions
3 oz. wild yam root	*Dioscorea villosa*	Lessens inflammation; balances hormones
3 oz. chasteberry	*Vitex agnus-castus*	Balances the hormone progesterone
2 oz. red clover flower	*Trifolium pratense*	Nutritious; has estrogenlike effects
1 oz. dong quai root	*Angelica sinensis*	Has estrogenlike effects; improves circulation; helps immunity
1 oz. licorice root	*Glycyrrhiza glabra*	Moistening; lessens inflammation; helps immunity

Ten ounces will last thirty days. Combine these herbal extracts. Take 1 teaspoon in 1 cup water in the morning and evening. If you are sensitive to licorice, increase wild yam to 4 ounces.

Dried Herbs	Botanical Names	Actions
3 oz. wild yam root	*Dioscorea villosa*	Lessens inflammation; balances hormones
2 oz. chasteberry seed	*Vitex agnus-castus*	Balances the hormone progesterone
1 1/2 oz. red clover flower	*Trifolium pratense*	Nutritious; has estrogenlike effects
1 oz. dong quai root	*Angelica sinensis*	Has estrogenlike effects; improves circulation; helps immunity
2 oz. licorice root	*Glycyrrhiza glabra*	Moistening; lessens inflammation; helps immunity
1/2 oz. rose petals	*Rosa* species	Lessen bleeding, infection

Fifteen ounces will last thirty days. Add 1/2 ounce of the mixture to 3 1/2 cups of boiling water in a teapot or container with a well-fitting lid. Omit rose petals if not organically grown. If you are sensitive to licorice, increase wild yam to 4 ounces. Let stand for fifteen minutes before straining. Drink 1 cup hot or cold three times a day. If you prefer, sip tea throughout the day or drink two larger glasses twice a day, making sure you drink 3 cups in a day.

Nutrition

Wise Food Choices
- Avoid excess coffee and alcohol.
- Soy foods, sprouted lentils, raw snow peas, and cooked green peas naturally increase your level of estrogen; use according to your personal taste. For a discussion of the effects of these foods, see the nutrition section in "Hot Flashes and Night Sweats" in Chapter 2, "Menopause."
- Add borage flowers, violet flowers, cucumber slices, and basil leaves in season to salads and sandwiches.

Supplements
- Flax seeds, 1 teaspoon daily. Soak in water twenty minutes; add to blended fruit drinks and salad dressings, or stir in cooked grains shortly before serving. You can also stir 1 to 2 teaspoons of powdered seeds in one or two glasses of water and drink the mixture immediately before or between meals. Or, if you prefer, take capsules as directed on labels.
- Vitamin E, 200 to 300 I.U. (international units) of vitamin E three times a day. After a week, reduce the vitamin E to 400 I.U. daily. More is not always

better—don't use more than 1,200 I.U. daily. If you have diabetes, hypertension, or a rheumatic heart condition, don't use more than 100 I.U. daily.
- Vitamin C, 1 gram three times a day, preferably with meals and vitamin E doses

In Addition

- Use essential oils with a reputation for aphrodisiac qualities as bath or massage oils. The use of lubricating aromatherapy for the vagina can help you get in touch with your body. A favorite combination is vitamin E combined with essential (volatile) oil of sandalwood, ylang ylang, or clary sage. To make your own massage or bath blend, place a total of 9 drops of one or all of the above essential oils in 1/2 ounce of vitamin E and 1/2 ounce of sesame, almond, or any other unheated vegetable oil. Stir 1/4 teaspoon into a bath or apply a few drops of the blend to fingertips; massage skin and genitalia. Lubricating herb mixtures shouldn't sting or irritate; don't use when skin is broken. If the oil does cause redness, you may have too strong a blend; try adding more vitamin E or vegetable oil. Also, rinse with plain cold water and wait a few days before trying again.
- Practice Kegel exercises (see box for "Kegels") five minutes a day to strengthen the muscles that make up the pelvic "floor."
- Sex stimulates secretion of moisture and germ-fighting enzymes in the mucous membranes of vaginal walls. If you experience discomfort in intercourse, or if vaginal dryness persists despite desire, your vagina may have an infection or may be thinning. For a fuller discussion of vaginal problems, see "Vaginal Thinning and Dryness" in Chapter 2, "Menopause."
- Don't douche much or at all. Among other things, it dries the vagina's mucous membranes, setting the scene for future irritation or infection. If you want to douche for relief of symptoms or other reasons, follow the directions below.

  To clear an itchy yeast infection or replenish vaginal membranes after repeated or severe vaginal infections, douche with toning and healing herbs such as lady's mantle, chamomile, sage, and licorice. Cover 1 ounce of any one or two (not all) with a pint of boiling water. After letting the mixture stand for fifteen minutes, strain and cool to a comfortable body temperature, and fill a douche bag with a simple bulb and applicator from the drugstore. Place the applicator tube into the first inch or two of the vaginal opening and gently squeeze the bulb to introduce the liquid. Or, if you do not have a douche bag, pour the mixture as a rinse over the vaginal folds while holding them open with the clean fingers of one hand. Douche no more than three days in a row and only if needed. After chronic infections, you can repeat the treatment every two weeks to help restore the integrity of the vaginal walls.

  For a fuller discussion on douching, see "Vaginal Thinning and Dryness" in Chapter 2, "Menopause."

- You can use herbal oils (not the same as essential or volatile oils) as frequently as needed. They help during intercourse to lubricate vaginal tissues, but they do more than reduce friction. St. John's wort and wild yam herb oils can lessen inflammation, heal raw places on the vaginal wall or cervix, and even be absorbed for mild, local hormonal benefits. These can be purchased, but some are more expensive than they need to be. If you are willing to fool around in the kitchen for two or three hours, you can make your own milder but effective, affordable vaginal salve or cream (see box for "More Love Vaginal Salve").

Kegels

These exercises cost no money and require no classes. Even a few weeks of practice makes a difference. Like yoga, the more consistently and the more slowly you do these painless exercises, the better the effects. Kegels (which rhymes with "bagels") are very safe and help all women. If you cannot hold urine when you laugh, sneeze, strain, or jump up and down, you need to do Kegels. Among other benefits, they help keep in a healthy baby whose mother has had a miscarriage and has borderline muscle tone. More universal is their effect on bladder and vaginal tone, helping women with urinary incontinence.

Kegels strengthen the muscles that make up the pelvic "floor" and add good blood flow. The pelvis is like a big basin or fruit bowl, with openings at the bottom that we control through muscle tone. Two pairs of symmetrical muscles that look like flower parts or butterfly wings hold your precious insides . . . well, inside. The two *pubococcygeus* muscles stretch from the pubic bone in front to the tailbone (coccyx) in back, like a mirror image, one on each side of the central urethra, the vaginal opening, and anus. Another pair are the *coccygeus* muscles, which connect the tailbone in back to the bones at the right and left sides of the pelvic basin. External pelvic muscles and structures reinforce both pairs. The perineum, which lies between your vaginal opening and the anus, is like a band that stretches from this center out to the right and left, connecting to the sides of the pelvic basin like an arched rainbow.

The pelvic floor also contains two sphincters. A sphincter is like a donut of muscle: If you clench it you can stop things from passing in or out. We have one muscle sphincter around the urethra and vagina and another around the anus. To feel which muscles these are, try an experiment. Sit on the toilet when you are passing a stream of urine. Tighten the muscles to stop the stream of urine. Let it go. Stop it again. You have just done two Kegels!

Now that you know from the experiment which muscles to "feel," repeat this tightening and letting go when you are not passing urine. Repeat and count Kegels in groups of ten, fifteen groups of four, or whatever numbers you like and feel best doing. Hold for longer or increase the number of repetitions at your own pace. You can do Kegels for any reason and at any time: standing at the sink making dinner, during intercourse, sitting in your car at a stoplight, standing in line, chatting on the phone. Not only will these exercises improve muscle tone when repeated frequently, but they also can improve orgasms, prevent complications of pregnancy (from hemorrhoids to miscarriage), and help the recovery of vaginal tone after delivery.

More Love Vaginal Salve

Fill a clean, dry, wide-mouth glass pint jar with 3 ounces of dried herb (2 ounces wild yam, 1 ounce St. John's wort). Pour in about 6 to 7 ounces of your choice of oil—for example, green, unfiltered, unheated olive oil, barely scented sweet almond oil, or safflower. Use enough oil to completely cover the herb. You should be able to barely stir to the bottom of the jar with a table knife or wooden chopstick. To prevent contamination, wipe the edges of the jar clean and dry before fitting on a tight lid. Leave in a warm location for ten days—on "low" in a crock pot away from the reach of small children, or place the jar in a pot half full of warm water and set it in an oven heated only by the pilot light, on a sunny windowsill, or on top of a water heater. The usual precaution about keeping herbal preparations away from heat and light doesn't apply here. In fact, it is the low heat that draws the herb into the oil, but without getting the oil hot enough to turn it rancid.

After ten days or so, filter out the oil from the herb in muslin or cheesecloth. It will take a little hand-wringing over a colander or bowl, so wear an apron. Discard the oily herb. Put strained herb oil into an enameled or stainless-steel saucepan over the lowest heat possible; melt in equal amounts of coconut oil and cocoa butter—for example, 1 ounce strained herb oil, 1 ounce coconut oil, 1 ounce cocoa butter. As an option, you may want to also add beeswax to add stability and thickness to your salve: Use 1/8 ounce (about the size of a walnut) for every ounce of oil.

To predict the consistency your salve will be when it cools and solidifies, dip a metal spoon in the oily mixture while it is warm liquid and refrigerate the spoon for five to ten minutes. After checking how the cooled mixture feels, add more of what's needed according to your preference: Oil makes it more liquid, cocoa butter makes it soft but solid at room temperature, and beeswax makes it the most solid. Redo the spoon test as you need to. It may take sixty to ninety minutes for a larger amount (4 to 6 ounces) to cool down and solidify completely at room temperature.

Even at this point you can decide what consistency you like. If it is too solid or too liquid, remelt as needed over the lowest possible heat source, such as a pan of steaming hot water. Make sure the salve jar is tightly closed so water cannot splash into it. Water and oil don't mix, especially in this recipe. When you are satisfied with its consistency, pour the liquid salve into a clean jar with a close-fitting lid.

Note: The rubber seals on canning jars containing oils go goopy and become discolored after a while, but this rarely hurts the oil if you keep checking and changing to fresh lids every few months. Plain metal lids that fit well are even better.

Congratulations—you have made an herbal salve! Use a teaspoon at a time for daily moisturizing or whenever "more love" is needed. You may want to experiment with other combinations after trying the basic recipe a couple of times.

Fibroids

Fibroids are benign growths. The term usually refers to fibrous growths of the uterus. They commonly occur in three places: in the wall of the uterine muscle, inside the uterus, or protruding from the uterine wall into the abdomen. Uterine tissue is estrogen sensitive; that is, the surfaces of its cells have receptors that are stimulated by circulating estrogen. An excess of estrogen stimulates the overgrowth and thickening of uterine tissue, eventually producing a fibroid. High levels of human growth hormone (HGH) can also trigger the growth of fibroids, so they may increase in late pregnancy.

Fibroids may remain small and unnoticed. Most will shrink or disappear after menopause when estrogen levels naturally go down. They can, however, grow large enough before menopause to cause damage, especially if they obstruct other structures or rupture and hemorrhage (causing internal bleeding). These serious conditions mainly happen if fibroids go untreated by natural therapies or conventional medical treatment.

Women with fibroids who are getting closer to menopause are often told they ought to have a hysterectomy, though this is not as worthwhile as previously believed. The presence of fibroids does not automatically mean that cancer will occur sooner or later or that they will block the intestines, threaten pregnancy, or cause anemia through heavy blood loss. Their size and severity, not their existence per se, determines their negative impact. Indeed, it is probable that at least one out of five adult women in the Western world have some bumps and knobs on their wombs. The American Medical Association reported in 1986 and again in 1988 that, according to second opinions from physicians within the conventional medical establishment, one-half of the seven hundred thousand hysterectomies annually performed in the United States, usually intended to remove uterine fibroids, were unnecessary.

If you can wait for the Change, the natural drop in estrogen at that time will allow the fibroids to shrink. Meanwhile, you can improve your quality of life in a number of ways.

Fibroids respond well to changes in nutrition as well as other therapies. If they are causing you discomfort, the first step is to decrease the common foods in your diet that worsen pain and create excess estrogen. For instance, eating less protein, especially animal products with high fat content, is a good way to start decreasing excess hormones. Using less salt provides other health benefits to the bones and heart. Second, gaining physical fitness improves pelvic circulation and uterine muscle tone. Third, you may wish to try herbal remedies that are known to speed the natural processes that shrink fibroids. These are just three of the numerous alternative methods available that may help you balance your health before you consider surgery.

Herbal Medicine

The following hormone-balancing tonics assist the menopausal process in decreasing estrogen-dependent fibroids. Combined with alteratives (cleansing herbs for altering chronic conditions), these tonics promote the body's own methods of lowering excess estrogen. Some of the herbs they contain also have an observed effect of helping with inflammation, sluggish pelvic circulation, and lymphatic drainage. The astringent or toning herbs here shrink the fibrous lumps and seal the muscle walls against infection or inflammation to promote a healthy womb. The herbs combine several overlapping actions that help return overgrowths of fibrous tissue to a healthier state, perhaps even to a perfect form.

REWEAVE ELIXIR

Extracts	Botanical Names	Actions
4 oz. wild yam root	*Dioscorea villosa*	Balances hormones; anti-inflammatory
4 oz. chasteberry seed	*Vitex agnus-castus*	Lowers excess estrogen; slows growth of fibroids
2 oz. sarsaparilla root	*Smilax ornata*	Supports hormone balance; improves lymphatic flow
2 oz. calendula flower	*Calendula officinalis*	Stimulates liver, immune, and lymph functions
2 oz. yarrow flower	*Achillea millefolium*	Tones tissue; lessens excessive bleeding

Fourteen ounces will last thirty to forty-five days depending on need. Combine these extracts. The dose is 1/2 teaspoon to 1 tablespoon (3 teaspoons) of the combination, diluted in an 8-ounce cup of liquid, three times a day.

REWEAVE TEA

Dried Herbs	Botanical Names	Actions
4 oz. wild yam root	*Dioscorea villosa*	Balances hormones; anti-inflammatory
4 oz. chasteberry seed	*Vitex agnus-castus*	Lowers excess estrogen; slows growth of fibroids
2 oz. sarsaparilla root	*Smilax ornata*	Supports hormone balance; improves lymphatic flow
2 oz. calendula flower	*Calendula officinalis*	Stimulates liver, immune, and lymph functions
2 oz. yarrow flower	*Achillea millefolium*	Tones tissue; lessens excessive bleeding

Fourteen ounces will last two weeks. Steep 1 ounce of this tea mixture in 4 cups of boiling water for twenty minutes, covered. Strain and drink 1 cup four times daily. The volume of water is itself cleansing and moisturizing. Be sure to empty the bladder before bed, however; drinking liquid late at night may interrupt sleep for a trip to the bathroom. The herbs will not aggravate night sweats if a woman with fibroids is already experiencing this other symptom of decreased estrogen. If night sweats are a problem, especially if they aggravate loss of sleep and fatigue, add 3 ounces motherwort. The bitter flavor is worth the benefits.

Whether you use tea or extract, continue for a minimum of one month before reducing the daily amount to 2 cups tea or two doses of extract. To safely double the dosage and avoid taking too much alcohol, which can occur if you are using the extract, drink both tea and extract. You can take one or both versions of this formula for another month or longer, until your body has reached a satisfying response to the herbs.

If after three to six months you do not experience a noticeable improvement—less pressure in the lower abdomen, more normal bleeding cycles, or confirmation of smaller fibroids by a health-care provider—switch to "Womb Rhythm"; see "Irregular Cycles" in Chapter 2, "Menopause." This formula is also recommended for fibroids complicated by heavy bleeding or spotting between cycles. You may want to ask your care provider for more information and take steps to rule out potential dangers associated with menopausal bleeding problems.

Fibroids also cause lower back pain and a dragging sensation or pressure that slows down a woman at the same time the chronic pain makes her feel depressed. There is help. Given time, nature's pain remedies are mild but heal deeply. Still, if you have any doubt that the herbs are helping, it is always wise to rule out other causes of back pain.

Nutrition

Wise Food Choices
- Eat more leafy, green vegetables: two to four servings a day, raw, steamed, or in soups. Vary according to individual preference, weather, seasonal availability, and your level of activity.
- Eat four servings a week of yellow and orange vegetables (carrots, squash, and the like).
- Eat whole grains, especially rice, three times a week.
- Avoid dairy (all milk products) for a minimum of three months.
- Avoid animal fats.

Supplements
- Fiber, especially flax seeds or psyllium husks, as directed on product labels. Fiber helps reduce congestion in the lower back, which can aggravate pain or pressure caused by fibroids.

In Addition
- Exercise brings improved circulation to the pelvis, delivering nutrients to the uterus as it heals itself. Also, activity decreases tension and helps the whole body (liver metabolism, especially) to balance hormones.
- External herbal therapies. There are several excellent options, three of which are listed here. Try *just one at a time*, choosing the one that appeals most. You can alternate their use if you wish, and you don't have to do all three.

- Castor oil packs. This external remedy is effective for some women but not for others, depending on the size of the fibroids, how slowly or quickly they are growing, and how consistently a woman applies them. See the directions in "Decline of Fertility," earlier in this chapter.
- Ginger compress. Place a handful of grated fresh ginger root in a cheesecloth and squeeze out the juice into 1 gallon of very hot water. Do not boil the water or you will lose the volatile power of the ginger. Dip a cotton hand towel into the ginger water, wring it out tightly, and apply it to the whole abdominal or lower back area. It should be very hot but not uncomfortably so. A second dry towel can be placed on top to reduce heat loss. Apply a fresh, hot ginger towel every two or three minutes until the skin becomes red but not uncomfortably hot. You can use a ginger compress daily for as long as a month before you reevaluate your progress.
- Poke root compress. You can apply 1/4 to 1/2 ounce of heated poke root tincture in a wash cloth as a hot compress to the area for four hours to overnight. To keep it hot that long, cover the compress with a heating pad or hot-water bottle. As an alternative, a strong decoction (2 ounces dried poke root to 8 ounces simmering water for fifteen minutes) makes a fine poultice; use the warmed pulp and tea together. If fresh grated poke root is available (check with an herb gardener; we're always trying to get rid of some), use 1/2 to 1 ounce with sufficient hot water to make a poultice. Use this nightly up to one month before reevaluation.

Whole-Body Effects of Premenopause

Whenever signs and symptoms of pre- or perimenopause are complicated or severe enough to demand professional attention, the cause may be a hormonal imbalance unrelated to estrogen or progesterone. Hormonal levels may fluctuate from the way the pancreas controls blood sugar, the adrenal glands' response to stress and immunity, thyroid changes affecting metabolism, and complex endocrine effects on sleep, mood, and the state of your nerves. To give just one example, several "menopausal" symptoms, such as moodiness, weight gain, low energy, and change in cycle could be attributed just as well to undiagnosed hypothyroidism, or low thyroid function.

The possibilities can be discomfiting, so if you don't know whether your periods and moods are changing because of menopause or a medical condition, see a nurse-practitioner, midwife, or other experienced female health-care provider, and talk with other women. If it's your style, read the relevant paragraphs in a dictionary of symptoms. Weight gain, changes in skin texture, unexpected desires—all have a few common causes. But don't blindly accept the opinions of others regarding causes and a diagnosis if they do not ring true. You know yourself better than anyone else, and you are the person who can best know how to balance your body's systems.

To achieve balance within, you will need to experiment and try some different herbal combinations. Although it may seem an odd comparison, the process is much like balancing a tire on a car. As every woman who has changed a tire knows, each of the lugnuts (four huge bolts) must be tightened only a little at a time, but not in logical progression around the wheel. If you completely tighten a bolt before going on to the next, by the time all four are tightened, the wheel will have twisted just enough to be off balance. We must do a little here, a little there, switching back and forth, not necessarily in logical order, turning the bolts a little more, until every bolt in the circle can be tightened with just one more turn of the wrench. The properly balanced wheel rolls smoothly along the ground without wobbling.

Balancing complex health concerns through natural therapy is similar. The goal is to reestablish hormonal balance by correcting each hormonal center gradually, not by treating each separate symptom in turn. The following herbs are taken up by the body and used as needed. This is not a concept accepted by conventional Western medicine; this is Western herbal medicine. The hormonal tonic herbs help the liver, digestion, circulation, or nerves as well as support balanced endocrine function. This slow but sure process avoids many of the side effects caused when herbs are taken in large doses to combat symptoms, allowing each woman's own body to regulate itself and establish its natural hormonal balance as soon as possible. No matter what seems a little "off balance," you can safely take the following combinations to balance the entire wheel of self-regulation.

Herbal Medicine

FULL CIRCLE

Extracts	Botanical Names	Actions
2 oz. bladderwrack seaweed	*Fucus vesiculosus*	Nutritive; helps balance thyroid function
3 oz. Siberian ginseng root	*Eleutherococcus senticosus*	Increases ability to cope with stress
2 oz. hawthorn flower, berry	*Crataegus monogyna*	Protects heart, blood vessels under stress
2 oz. wild yam root	*Dioscorea villosa*	Provides whole-body hormonal benefits
2 oz. St. John's wort herb	*Hypericum perforatum*	Lifts depression; helps nerves, immunity
1 oz. suma root	*Pfaffia paniculata*	Lessens sugar cravings; improves immune response

Twelve ounces will last thirty days. Combine these herbal extracts. Take 1 teaspoon in 1 cup water in the morning and at midday. A third teaspoon may be taken early in the evening before dinner if you are feeling a lot of stress or need to curb overeating caused by emotional challenges. Sometimes whole pieces or powder of suma root are hard to find on store shelves. In that case, add another 1/2 ounce each of St. John's wort and wild yam.

FULL CIRCLE TEA

Dried Herbs	Botanical Names	Actions
5 oz. Siberian ginseng root	*Eleutherococcus senticosus*	Increase ability to cope with stress
5 oz. wild yam root	*Dioscorea villosa*	Provides whole-body hormone benefits
3 oz. hawthorn flower, berry	*Crataegus monogyna*	Protects heart, blood vessels under stress
1 oz. licorice root	*Glycyrrhiza glabra*	Moisture, flavor; reduces sweet cravings
1 oz. sage leaf	Salvia officinalis	Aids digestion, benefits hormone balance

Fifteen ounces will last thirty days. Add 1/2 ounce of the mixture to 3 1/3 cups boiling water in a teapot or container with a well-fitting lid. Let stand for thirty minutes before straining. Drink 1 cup hot or cold three times a day. If you prefer, sip tea throughout the day or drink two larger glasses twice a day, making sure you drink 3 cups a day. Hawthorn berries are easier to find than the more medicinal flowers and leaves, so you may need to start with the berries and ask your supplier to place a special order for the flowers and leaves. If you are sensitive to licorice, replace it with 1 ounce fennel seeds.

Nutrition

Wise Food Choices

Eating well most of the time is an important way to stabilize your changing neurochemical soup. This does not mean overeating gourmet dishes; it means, rather, enjoying smaller amounts of concentrated or nutrition-packed whole foods in season.

- Avoid packaged convenience foods, refined flour, sugar and junk food, additives (especially monosodium glutamate [MSG]), and table salt.
- Eat two fresh pieces of organic fruit in season, each and every day. True dietary intolerance to fruit is not as common as people think. If you are avoiding it for that reason or because of problems with yeast or a lack of interest in

boring supermarket fruit "look-alikes," make a special effort and choose local, fresh organic fruit in season. Raw fruit (and edible seeds) offer many benefits that promote healing: vitamins, minerals, acids, moisture, fiber, complex carbohydrates, protein mixed with enzymes, and essential fatty acids.

- Have at least three vegetables a day: one red vegetable, one yellow, and one green.
- Use 1 to 4 ounces per week of any edible seaweed: kelp, dulse, sea fronds, and others, available packaged at natural-food stores and often accompanied by recipes for soup stock, stir-fried vegetables, and noodle dishes. Edible seaweeds are often ignored in modern Western diets, but they specifically assist endocrine balance. In fishing communities on the coasts of Wales, Japan, and the North American Pacific, small servings of a wide variety of seaweed were traditionally and regularly used to prevent the ills of middle-aged people. Though sea vegetables contain sea salt, they also have all the minerals of the sea and other cofactors that help us readily use and excrete salt. If you have special sodium restrictions, check with your health-care provider; you may be able to try small servings (1/4 ounce dried seaweed prepared as directed in package-label recipes or as desired).

Supplements

- Kelp, 2 tablets with meals once a day, though all tablets are a poor substitute for delicious sea vegetables

In Addition

- Exercise, especially if you think you are too tired to do it.
- Walk twenty minutes a day, perhaps at lunch with a friend.

Premenopause may take you by surprise. Sometimes it catches us unaware and unprepared because we are focused on other health issues or life challenges during the years preceding middle age. But for us today, embracing all the changes of menopause can be, as it is in many cultures, the beginning of true wisdom. Achieving wisdom does not mean acting old; it means acting with the power that knowledge and experience bring. Now, as we reach the end of one millennium and begin another, more women are reaching back to prehistory for the tools that optimum health requires today. Herbal remedies to strengthen us along our journey are one way to open doors, the other side of which we have only dreamed. But knowledge of ancient and modern tools is not enough. We can know something full well and not act upon our knowledge. To be empowered demands action, even if it is simply the internal steps taken inside ourselves. Only when we take action to ensure our own well-being are we free to respond to the unpredictable challenges of this hormonal rite of initiation.

Chapter 2

MENOPAUSE

The word *menopause,* a combination of two Greek words—*men* and *pausis*—literally means a pause in menses. This life stage is unique to humans: no other animals go through it. Also known as the "Change of Life," or the "Change," menopause occurs when our ovaries have stopped releasing the eggs they contained at birth. A strict definition of *menopause* is a complete cessation of menstrual periods. In common usage, however, it refers to the whole time when a woman's cycle is changing (the more formal term is *perimenopause,* and it is also called the *climacteric*).

The range for starting natural menopause is as wide as thirty-six to sixty years of age; in the vast majority of women, it begins at about fifty-one. Unless you get a blood test for elevated FSH (follicle-stimulating hormone), which most women don't bother with unless they're having severe symptoms, only in hindsight can you be diagnosed as having gone through menopause. The average length of the menopausal transition is just over a year but can last for several years. After twelve to twenty-four months without menstrual bleeding or pregnancy, a woman is considered to be "done" with menopause. But even this is not an absolute: Some women are surprised by an erratic return of the menstrual cycle when they change their diets, fall in love, or start taking herbs. Some women joke that the word *menopause* means there are "many pauses" in their blood flow before it is over.

Menopause is signaled by some common signs and symptoms, but women experience them in varying intensity. Depending on which statistics one reads, as many as 80 percent of women have a fairly normal menopause, which may include symptoms such as hot flashes, night sweats, and irregular cycles; 10 percent have no signs at all; and 10 percent have some kind of severe health breakdown related to menopause. In addition, minor health problems or lurking constitutional weaknesses, such as poor circulation or a tendency toward arthritis, may surface during menopause.

As they enter this new stage of life, women experiencing menopause's physiological changes also may identify new emotional and spiritual challenges in their lives and reevaluate their previous ways of living and their cultural beliefs. Menopause is unsettling enough, but it also requires us to fend off negative social beliefs about what it is and what it means to a woman, challenging us to confront Western society's perceptions about aging, about older women, about our preoccupation with youth, and to accept this new stage of life as a natural transformation. In cultures where there is a greater respect for elders, menopause is considered a natural rite of passage and as less of a "problem."

Added to all these concerns is the notion—held by ourselves and others—that anything that is natural, including menopause, should be a snap. We're all familiar with this myth: Somewhere out in the world are women who always eat right, always stay in emotional equilibrium, and sail through menopause without trauma or need for medication. This is the easiest notion about menopause to dispel: Believe it—there is no such perfect person on the face of the Earth! Though some women have no problems, if you do have difficulty, that does not mean you are somehow inadequate or blameworthy. Certainly we can be more forgiving to ourselves than that.

On the deepest level, women in menopause can find their new prime, though to do so they must allow their old selves to pass away and discover anew who they are. There is an awareness of the mortality of one's physical body, which can be a liberating or a frightening revelation depending on a woman's belief system. It is not surprising that most women feel depressed or uncertain during these years. We may ponder the meaning of our lives thus far or feel overwhelmed by the possible paths still ahead of us before our ultimate physical passing. Thoughts of death are natural; contemplation of suicide may occur. Just because a woman has these feelings does not mean she's "crazy" or abnormal. But we need to talk about our feelings with each other. Sharing experiences and feelings with good friends or seeking professional counseling may free you from your private fears as you go through this challenging transition. As you face the challenge of menopause, it's important to keep it in perspective: Menopause is not a disease requiring treatment; it is a natural biological change.

Above all, we need to realize that after a temporary period of trial, whether mild or intense, every woman can enter the second half of her life with a wisdom and dignity no maiden can match. Given all the challenges presented by menopause, a woman's choices to help with this transition range from the most simple remedies (such as rest and mild herbs) to the more complex, including hormone replacement therapy and surgery. To choose well, a woman of power simply needs to understand all her options.

The rest of this chapter explores common menopausal health conditions and the use of herbs to encourage a positive menopausal transformation. For centuries, simple and safe plant remedies have made the outward signs of this internal change more agreeable. In addition, general tips on whole-food nutrition for all the specific conditions discussed in this chapter can be found in the "Herbs and Nutrition in Menopause" section that follows.

Herbs and Nutrition in Menopause

Gaining five to ten pounds at menopause is natural because nature knows what is coming and how to protect us. The extra fat helps cushion the drop of estrogen because fat cells make a tiny amount of estrogen. A lot more fat is not helpful, however; nor is severe weight loss. Fad diets, obsessive aerobics, and starvation are antagonistic to the vibrancy that can be yours when you relax into the "Change." A healthy weight and a steady routine of physical activity should be the goal. Without going to extremes, women *can* control their weight and appearance as they change during menopause.

The wild card determining your ease or difficulty with this rite of passage may hinge on your attitude. Eating wisely may break a few calorie-counting rules and requires you to keep an open mind. For instance, it's perfectly fine to eat some nuts and seeds because the teaspoon or so added to a salad or to other dishes really isn't that fattening. Your body does not look as it did when you were sixteen, nor should it: You are a fully mature woman. Try seeing yourself with loving, not critical eyes, letting out the hidden feminine power within.

A varied, unrefined whole-food diet based on grains, fresh fruit, and vegetables in season may help ease the transition. Especially nourishing are wheat germ (for vitamin E), yogurt (for low-fat energy, calcium, and strong intestinal flora), apricots (for iron), garlic (to lessen our risk of heart disease), and sprouts (for essential fatty acids to protect nerves, quick energy, and some safe, food-based estrogen). Women who have an easier menopause tend to avoid excess protein and phosphorous-rich foods, red meat, refined flour, sugar and junk food, additives, added salt, smoking, alcohol, and caffeine (including chocolate and many brands of diet sodas). A temporary break from hot spices is also helpful.

Foods rich in plant estrogens, or phytoestrogens (mild vegetable hormones with effects like natural estrogen in humans), are highly recommended during menopause. In a British study, twenty-three menopausal women ate foods rich in phytoestrogens—soy flour, red clover sprouts, and flax seeds in an amount equal to 10 percent of daily calories—for two weeks. During that time period, the degree of vaginal cell maturation (a sign of estrogen levels) went up 40 percent, causing the researchers to theorize that estrogen pills would be obsolete if women ate these foods. These findings were corroborated by an Australian study in which women averaging fifty-nine years ate 45 grams (1 1/2 ounces) of soy flour every day for two weeks, then 25 grams (about an ounce) of linseed (flax seed) meal daily for two weeks, then 10 grams (1/3 ounce) of red clover sprouts. Again, vaginal cell maturation showed significant improvement that lasted another two weeks after the women stopped using these foods.

Eating well most of the time is a strong way of stabilizing your body's ever-changing neurochemical soup. The following lists are not absolute, but they do provide guidelines about foods to avoid and foods to increase in your regular eating patterns.

The "Low" to "No" List

- Fats, especially animal fats such as cheese and red meat. Aim to eat less than 30 to 40 grams of fat a day, or less than 10 to 30 percent of your daily calories in fat.
- Excess protein, beyond 10 to 20 percent of your daily caloric intake, or 50 grams.

- Packaged convenience foods
- Refined flour, sugar, junk food
- Additives (especially monosodium glutamate [MSG])
- Table salt, including excess "natural" sodium in tamari, soy sauce, and similar items
- Alcohol (especially red wine)
- Caffeine (including chocolate and sodas, diet sodas)
- Nicotine
- In addition, avoid overdependence on phosphorous-rich foods such as a "mono-diet" of legumes, yellow corn, nuts, and parsnips because phosphorous and calcium compete for the honor of being in your body. Eating too much phosphorous in an unbalanced diet diminishes calcium. However, the phytosterols of many legumes (peas, beans) and the essential fatty acids of raw nuts and seeds (almonds, sesame) have tremendous benefits for menopausal women. As with most things in life, the key here is moderation and common sense.

The "Yes" List

- Whole grains (brown rice, buckwheat, whole wheat with bran and wheat germ, whole oats, other grains)
- Fresh fruit in season, organic if possible
- Red, yellow, and green vegetables
- Various root vegetables (carrots, beets, burdock in soup, turnips, rutabaga, raw jicama in salads)
- Leafy green vegetables, organic if possible—all kinds, to taste
- Iron from food sources is more easily assimilated and will not cause constipation, unlike many iron supplements. Good choices include unsulphured dried apricots, soaked a few hours in spring water (making them easier to digest), raw pumpkin seeds (1/2 tablespoon sprinkled on salads), and blackstrap molasses. If you are not used to the taste of molasses, try a little, which tastes better than a lot at once. A very healthful breakfast is old-fashioned oatmeal porridge or another hot cereal served with a teaspoon of molasses and a few golden or brown raisins, to taste. Instant or microwaved starch-in-five-minutes-style oatmeal is not a brilliant example of Western civilization's progress; leave it out. You can make real oatmeal almost as quickly: Organic rolled oats take only five to fifteen minutes once the water is boiling.
- For good-quality essential fatty acids (helpful to immunity, nerves, and hormonal balance), enzymes (for overall metabolism and especially good digestion of proteins), and easily digested protein, try the liberal use of sprouted seeds and legumes. You can find sprouts at natural-food stores, or you can purchase dried seeds and sprout them at home. Soy, sunflower, aduki, fenugreek, onion, and other live green sprouts provide an array of vitamins, minerals, phytoestrogens, and chlorophyll to sweeten the belly and the breath.
- A little plain, live yogurt is fine if you can tolerate dairy foods. The dairy question is explored more fully in "Osteoporosis."

- Diuretic foods that help prevent water retention and bloating are freshly grated cabbage, cucumber, pineapple, parsley, watermelon, and cantaloupe. Cabbage, broccoli, and brussels sprouts have health benefits including cancer prevention, but eaten in excess they may worsen digestive gas, so use them to the extent you find best for your needs. Vitamin B_6, also a diuretic, is needed even more than usual when women have taken the Pill, because after three years of use, the Pill decreases assimilation of B_6. Low B_6 is also associated with diabetes, while the whole B complex is associated with good blood-sugar stability.
- The B vitamin complex (found in whole grains, legumes, dairy, animal products) ensures healthy nerves. One can get enough from nonanimal sources with a balanced whole-food diet.
- When optimizing liver function is important, as with hepatitis, a past history of substance abuse, or other liver damage, add the herb milk thistle to the diet (1 tablespoon seeds daily). These nutty-tasting, rice-size brown seeds can be freshly ground in a coffee grinder and added to foods such as salad dressings, protein drinks, fruit smoothies, and soups or sprinkled over cooked grains. Milk thistle helps protect regenerating liver cells. Larger amounts can be taken as a supplement if needed.
- A word about the tendency to overuse multivitamins and supplements: In general, don't rely on tablets for your basic nutrition; they are hard to digest and may not be assimilated well. Worse, in my opinion, overuse of supplements may teach the body to get rusty in some of its functions; sometimes the body will only perform certain digestive processes if enzyme supplements are chewed with food. Try choosing foods that you enjoy and that supply the basic nutrition you need, and leave the supplements for only those genuine deficiencies that satisfying nutritional foods cannot resolve.

Cardiovascular Disease

In recent years, estrogen's protection against diseases of the cardiovascular system (CVS) has been big news, with the risk of cardiovascular disease said to be related to a woman's level of estrogen. Though this is not the whole story, conventional medicine and popular media have repeatedly told women that we catch up with men in terms of heart attacks, strokes, and other heart disease at menopause. Now new studies are questioning the cardiovascular benefits of hormone replacement therapy and estrogen replacement therapy (discussed more fully in Chapter 3).

With or without hormones complicating the scene, medical researchers have not yet uncovered all the facts about heart disease. Yes, serum cholesterol and triglycerides (blood fats) do go up after the Change. The drop in estrogen around this age is assumed to be the single major cause, and higher blood fat levels and low estrogen do occur together. But these two body changes by themselves do not lead to myocardial infarctions (heart attacks), especially if a woman was not at risk for a heart attack anyway (see "Risk Factors for Cardiovascular Disease"). Because estrogen has been studied as an isolated hormone, its effects may have been taken out of context. The body has complex ways of staying in balance. In menopause a woman's body reacts to changes in estrogen levels, yet menopause is more than a single effect of any one chemical, even ones as potent as hormones. We do know that estrogen affects the cardiovascular system by increasing heart-protecting HDLs (high-density lipoproteins, or "good" fats) that counteract LDLs (low-density lipoproteins, "bad," cholesterol-laden fats). Meanwhile, estrogen stimulates more than four hundred types of cells that have estrogen receptors, so giving it as a replacement in menopause affects more than heart and blood.

Progesterone's role in postmenopausal heart disease is also unclear. Blamed for lowering HDL, progesterone can also help us by lowering blood fats. Women still have some progesterone throughout the Change, so in the past, conventional medical researchers have assumed that to lower the risks of heart disease related to menopause women need to be dosed with estrogen. But today fewer women are taking estrogen by itself because it carries with it an increased risk of cancers (uterine lining, endometrial, and perhaps others). The conventional medical opinion is that if a woman no longer has her uterus, it is okay to prescribe estrogen alone for preventing CVS risks, but estrogen does increase risks of other health concerns including breast cancer. The combination of estrogen and progesterone (HRT), which is considered safer, is commonly prescribed to women who have not had a hysterectomy. Nevertheless, studies do not agree that HRT gives the same cardiovascular benefits as estrogen alone. The picture remains confused. One study of women of the same age, some premenopausal and others in menopause, showed they had different estrogen levels but the same cardiovascular risks. It appears that the presence or absence of estrogen in menopause is not the biggest cause of women's higher heart attack rates after menopause.

Risk Factors for Cardiovascular Disease

High-fat diet	High salt intake
Smoking	Diabetes
Family history	Lack of exercise
High blood pressure	Emotional or physical stress or trauma
Obesity	High cholesterol, especially high levels of low-density lipoproteins (LDLs)

In reality, postmenopausal heart disease may have more to do with unhealthy lifestyles than the lack of estrogen. Indeed, postmenopausal heart attacks have been on the rise since World War II, a period in which more women have been smoking, eating fast foods high in fats and salt, and working at full-time jobs outside the home. Heart problems in older women today are more likely due to weight, the ratio of HDL (good) to LDL (bad) fats, family history of heart problems, smoking, lifelong health, or recent patterns of nutrition and exercise. Add to this the effects of stress on the heart, and one can see that the problem of heart disease should not be explained away as a menopausal "lack" of estrogen.

Medicine already supports this idea, because it is well known that, for example, making common-sense changes in our diets and not smoking lower cardiovascular risks. Natural therapists suggest that in addition to adopting healthy habits, one may be able to lower heart attack risks another way: by making midlife the time for opening one's heart to what is, rather than pining for what is past. This Change of Life for both men and women requires a "change of heart"—new ways of coping with life's challenges for fulfillment at this age. We know a go-getter attitude or a stressful style of approaching life's ups and downs is part of the makeup of those most likely to suffer heart disease. A healing response to heart problems may be to change stressful work patterns, old patterns of eating and carousing, and feelings of hard-heartedness in an emotional relationship.

Some research suggests that menopausal symptoms are better balanced by giving progesterone rather than adding estrogen. This may explain why herbs found to be helpful for menopause do not all necessarily have estrogenic effects. Several traditional remedies for hot flashes and other menopausal symptoms instead promote the body's production of progesterone and related hormones.

A last note about heart health, fat, and hormones: When women in the Change are in anything resembling reasonable health, androgens (masculine sex hormones) are still present as part of the hormonal "soup." These are gradually changed into estrone (a type of estrogen) in the adrenal glands, in fat cells, and elsewhere. For this reason, maintaining a healthy, protective number of fat cells will naturally provide more estrone, which in turn means fewer problems from the loss of estrogen produced by the ovaries—a good argument for keeping a little cushion of body fat while maintaining fitness and against the obsessive overattention some women put on reducing to a fat-free, bone-thin, androgynous body type.

Herbal Medicine

The following herbal formulas help the entire cardiovascular system, especially for those women who are in higher-risk groups. While the herbs also help with hot flashes, they are specifically designed to strengthen blood vessels and heart muscle, normalize blood pressure, and improve circulation to the fingers and toes. They will not cause negative interactions with medication for high blood pressure and are safe for children or men to drink, too.

❦ ——————— CHANGE OF HEART CORDIAL ——————— ❦

Extracts	Botanical Names	Actions
4 oz. hawthorn leaf, flower, berry	*Crataegus* species	Safety relaxes blood vessels; lowers high blood pressure
2 oz. motherwort herb	*Leonurus cardiaca*	Lessens hot flashes; calms a pounding heart
2 oz. chasteberry seed	*Vitex agnus-castus*	Stabilizes hormone surges and declines
1 oz. black cohosh root	*Cimicifuga racemosa*	Hormone tonic; relaxes and nourishes nerves
1/2 oz. blackstrap molasses		Nutritive; provides iron without causing constipation
2 1/2 oz. black cherry juice concentrate		For taste; to harmonize strong herbal actions (available at natural-food stores)

Twelve ounces will last thirty days. Combine these herbal extracts. Take 1 teaspoon twice a day, diluted in 1 cup of water, juice, or any herb tea, in the morning and evening.

❦ ——————— CHANGE OF HEART TEA ——————— ❦

Dried Herbs	Botanical Names	Actions
2 oz. linden flower	*Tilia* species	Moistens, relaxes; tones blood vessels and nerves
2 oz. hawthorn flower, leaf	*Crataegus* species	Nourishes heart; stabilizes circulation
2 oz. hawthorn berry	*Crataegus* species	Nourishes heart; stabilizes circulation
1/2 oz. hibiscus flower	*Hibiscus sabdariffa*	For taste, cooling; nutritive
1 oz. peppermint leaf	*Mentha piperita*	Soothes digestion; for taste

Fifteen ounces will last thirty days. Put 1/2 ounce of the mixture and 3 1/2 cups of boiling water in a teapot or container with a well-fitting lid. Let stand for fifteen minutes before straining. Drink 1 cup hot or cold three times a day, either sipping the tea all day or drinking two large glasses twice a day. If you don't care for peppermint, replace it with either rosemary or raspberry leaves.

Nutrition

Wise Food Choices

- Eat smaller meals more often.
- Limit fats in the diet to 10 to 20 percent of total daily calories (not the 30 percent allowed by conventional dietitians or the 45 percent common in the American diet).
- If you choose to eat eggs, use them in moderation. Even in a low-fat diet, two to three nonfried eggs per week are fine. No matter how many commercials by egg and dairy lobbies you see, choose organic and free-range eggs. (Nonorganic eggs are loaded with hormones and chemicals. Free-range chickens that scratch around in organic soil for minerals, bugs, and grains produce healthier eggs and a healthier environment than caged, battery-operated hens fed antibiotics under commercial production techniques.)
- Increase intake of vitamin E for its antioxidant benefits and its role in helping older people cope with stress and aging. It occurs naturally in vegetable oils, eggs, unprocessed cereals, some fish and meat, and leafy vegetables. Sprouted seeds, besides being rich in essential fatty acids that nourish the skin and the immune system, provide vitamin E, enzymes, and readily digestible protein. Avocados, wheat germ, and flax seed are other food sources of vitamin E.
- Use healthy fats (HDLs) to help prevent cardiovascular disease. Omega-3 fatty acids are found in seafood; other helpful fatty acids are found in oats and dried beans (legumes), so enjoy oatmeal and split pea soup!
- One clove of raw or lightly steamed garlic a day is preventative for high cholesterol, hardened arteries, and other factors of heart disease. Women in higher-risk groups can eat more, up to three cloves a day. Even if you love garlic, you'll know you are at the upper limit of what your body can use if you start to get an upset stomach, in which case take a break from it or try less. If you can't take much garlic, try these alternatives: Add it finely chopped to steamed vegetables, soups, or rice during the last five to ten minutes of cooking. Add a handful of finely chopped parsley or a teaspoon of dried leaves, freshly crumbled between your palms, to the dish before eating. After dinner, sweeten your breath by nibbling on a few cardamom seeds. If you just can't eat garlic, deodorized capsules and tablets are available; take as directed on label. If these don't agree with you, don't worry about missing the benefits of garlic—it isn't the only way to help your heart.
- Increase fiber in the form of vegetables, fruit, and whole grains (for example, whole oats have more nutritional value and are cheaper than oat bran).
- Limit intake of caffeine, as it raises blood pressure, blood fats, and your risk of heart disease.

- Limit alcohol use; one glass of wine or beer with the evening meal may help some people lower their risk of heart disease, but for most people larger amounts over time increase the risk of cardiovascular disease and many other illnesses.
- Avoid animal fats from red meat, chicken, cheese, milk, and rich seafood. However, seafood is rich in Omega-3 fatty acids, helpful in preventing heart disease. If you choose to eat seafood, emphasize white or lean fish, which are lower in calories than lobster, crab, salmon, and sardines, all of which are high in fat. Fatty seafood is great for getting Omega-3; just don't eat it every day as a preventative therapy!
- Avoid hydrogenated or partially hydrogenated fats (margarine, many packaged foods, snack items).
- Avoid salt and monosodium glutamate (MSG). We get more than enough sodium in vegetables, grains, proteins, and whole foods. An excess of added table salt leads to water retention, high blood pressure, and other complaints.

Supplements
- If you have problems enjoying garlic, try deodorized capsules; take as directed on product labels.
- To quickly lower cholesterol, try fiber, especially psyllium, flax, or chia seeds. Mix 1 teaspoon powdered seeds in an 8-ounce glass of water (if soaked for any length of time, the seeds will form a gelatinous mixture). Or take them in capsules as directed on product labels, making sure to drink eight glasses of water during the day. If you do not drink this extra water, the fiber absorbs all your body's water, possibly creating some constipation. This is why cooked grains, legumes, or fresh whole vegetables, which contain the right amount of water for their fiber content, are better than fiber supplements in the long term.
- Omega-3 fatty acids are anti-inflammatory, decrease the risk of strokes, and lower blood fats. Several products are available; use as directed on labels.

In Addition
- Exercise according to your body type and favorite movements.
- Stop smoking. It is never too late, and it will do you a world of good.
- Meditate (see box for "Opening the Heart Meditation").

Osteoporosis

Osteoporosis, the depletion of calcium in our bones, is a big concern for women throughout menopause. Bones affected by this disease are porous and weakened and may lead to fractures, back pain, loss of height, and stooped posture. The condition is quite common; according to conventional medical publications severe osteoporosis is said to affect about 25 percent of postmenopausal women.

Opening the Heart Meditation

If you record this meditation, you may wish to leave a silent pause of thirty seconds or more where asterisks (*) appear. Find five minutes in a quiet spot and sit or lie in a comfortable position. Close your eyes for the meditation.

Count your breath evenly and slowly. * Now tune in to the beating of your heart. It is a drumbeat. Let it sound evenly and slowly with your breath. No other thoughts or feelings are allowed to interrupt your loving attention to your natural rhythmic heartbeat. In your mind's eye, you see or imagine your heart is not only red, but also green, like a garden. It is cool and moist, very tender. Some places in the garden of your heart are hot and strong, like a magnificent crimson rose, a passionate river of lava, capable of changing the world.

As you slowly stroll through your garden, you stop and admire the beauty and fragrance of the flowers bending over the path. At your feet are a few weeds sprouting here and there. You talk to them, saying you will change their physical form now. You find yourself easily uprooting the ones you can see. You recognize these weeds in your imaginary garden of the heart as the hard words spoken yesterday or an old envy, a missed joy. As you remove the weeds from the path winding through your inner landscape of emotions, name them if you can. When you have weeded enough for today, visualize yourself carrying the limp remains of the plants out of the garden, and place them where they may decompose into rich earth for tomorrow's flowers.

As you face your garden before leaving, you notice that the flowers have doubled since you last looked. Your dark thoughts have been freed. Sun and shadow dance in your heart.

Tune in to the beat of your heart once more. Count your breathing slowly and evenly. * When you feel ready, bring your full attention back to the place where you sit in silence.

Tending to this inner vision of your changing heart makes room for love, for both others and ourselves. In contemplation or in the physical realm, there is nothing like a little gardening, just five minutes here and there, to open one's heart.

As women go through menopause, the drop in estrogen affects the bones' ability to retain calcium. Up until menopause, estrogen has a stimulating effect on our body's bone-building activity throughout life. Around puberty, sudden increases of estrogen provide extra stimulation for growth spurts. Later, through our reproductive years, estrogen stimulates the continued formation of strong bones to pick up our growing children or to handle the mineral loss of menstruation. After our reproductive years, the decreased stimulation of bones by estrogen can be compensated for by continuing exercise and optimizing bone strength with all the factors in our control. Those that natural therapies can address follow in these pages.

You may not realize you are developing this condition because it occurs gradually at the cellular level. We all have two types of bone cells. The osteoblasts (bone-makers) are cells that take minerals from the bloodstream and use them to build concentric rings of strong bone. Their opposite twin cells, the osteoclasts (bone-*un*makers), are constantly taking away dense bone material and breaking it down to return minerals to the bloodstream. This natural and healthy process allows the bones to handle the body's constantly changing demand for minerals. We need calcium and other minerals in the blood for activities happening at the cellular level throughout the body. These activities include maintaining a steady heartbeat, keeping the kidneys' excretion of wastes in happy balance, and soothing our frazzled nerves. This exchange of minerals from bone to blood and from blood to bone ensures the bones are always in the process of being re-formed with new building materials.

Your level of physical activity provides stimulus for the osteoblasts, so that you make bones just as dense as your activity level demands. With movement, bones thicken the more they are used for a particular activity. This is the bones' natural response to body signals that they prepare for more of the same activity. Without regular body movement bones have no good reason to be strong. Inactivity, not a decline in estrogen, is your bones' enemy. While you sit reading this book, your bones have dissolved a little of their calcium strength to the bloodstream, for whatever purpose the body needs.

In fact, exercise is widely seen as a major way to prevent osteoporosis. According to a Massachusetts Medical Society report of a study by the *British Medical Journal* in 1987, aerobic exercise and muscle strengthening can increase bone density and improve general health in menopausal women. It's never too late to start, but the best effects are seen in women who begin regular moderate exercise at least by age thirty-five and continue beyond menopause.

Your exercise program should fit the level of your tolerance or fitness, and it should be a pleasurable discipline that can be done often. Anything that combines muscle contraction and the good effects of gravity's pull on your bones will help prevent bone loss, so good choices are walking, running, dancing, bicycling, and weight training. At the very least, keep your posture straight and walk a lot. It has been said that swimming is not weight-bearing, but pushing against the resistance of the water is an excellent start for women with weak joints or weight problems. Seek out support groups or friends with whom you actually enjoy exercising to make it fun.

Like exercise, estrogen stimulates the osteoblasts to turn calcium in the bloodstream into dense bone. This is why estrogen replacement has been presented to women as a treatment or prevention for osteoporosis. If you have a severe risk of osteoporosis, estrogen replacement probably will stimulate bone density, although by itself it is not the best method for ensuring healthy bones past menopause.

Taking estrogen within three years of menopause postpones *some* of the natural bone loss resulting from a drop in estrogen, so it is assumed, but not proven, that taking estrogen *sooner* will prevent osteoporosis and fractures. This assumption is not always borne out. All women with osteoporosis don't break their hips, and not all middle-aged or elderly women with fractures have a bone density problem. Some women with hip fractures have bone densities similar to those who don't break any bones. In general, osteoporosis studies do not consider other possible causes of broken bones in women: the isolation of greater numbers of single aging women, poverty among the elderly, public safety, or housing conditions.

In a 1988 Italian study of women with fibroids who were on medication to lower estrogen and other ovarian steroids, the women were tested for bone mineral content, bone density, and bone width. Despite lower estrogen no significant changes were seen in their bones. Although one study does not prove anything definitively, it does suggest that less estrogen does not *automatically* lead to brittle bones.

There is more to osteoporosis than the exercise and estrogen issues. Even without definitive proof about their efficacy, calcium supplements are widely recommended to middle-aged women for prevention of osteoporosis. Yet calcium is one of the most abundant, widely available minerals in whole foods, so we are not likely to be calcium deficient through diet. Do we automatically need to consume between 1 and 2 grams of calcium per day (an average dose of 1,200 to 1,500 milligrams), in addition to whatever is in our salad bowls? This high amount is still standard advice, whether from physicians, medical newspaper columnists, or some alternative health publications, whose advertisers make calcium or multimineral supplements.

Getting calcium from the food we eat is by far our best option. For most women, the calcium from many whole foods—called "bioavailable calcium"—is easily absorbed in the digestive process, which makes it "bioavailable." Some examples of calcium-rich vegetables include slightly bitter greens such as kale and chard, which also encourage healthy stomach acid, necessary for calcium assimilation. Many commercial calcium supplements, on the other hand, have an alkaline carrier (antacids) that neutralizes stomach acids, making calcium absorption far less likely. Taking larger amounts of supplements will not ensure better uptake. Besides, too much calcium can act like an alkaline chalk, interfering more seriously with acidic digestive juices. When these digestive secretions are the wrong pH, women can begin to have problems breaking down food, maintaining general immune resistance, and avoiding anemia. Another potential problem of excessive calcium supplementation is its effect on the kidneys, which clear the bloodstream when it is burdened with too much of this mineral. The kidneys excrete excess calcium via urine. Excess calcium can lead to urinary-tract problems, even kidney stones.

Calcium in the diet does not have to come from dairy products. In fact, nuts, seeds, and greens are more bioavailable sources of calcium and other nutrients for mature women than milk, cheese, antacids, or sugary colon cleansers. This is partially because we need vitamins and minerals that are in natural proportions, as found in many whole foods. Leafy vegetables and other nondairy sources of calcium also help protect our hearts and may improve our pain sensitivity, two things worsened by overdependence on animal products. Another concern with dairy products is the industry's use of antibiotic-laced cattle feeds and stimulating growth hormones.

Vegetable and nut sources of calcium are a greater part of diets in other parts of the world such as Asia, where women don't eat a lot of cheese, don't take calcium supplements, and don't have anything like our Western "epidemic" of osteoporosis. The Asian diet is traditionally lower than ours in meat and protein, while dairy is rarely eaten. Asian women eat half or less of the calcium load in their lives than Western women, and their bones are not thinning nearly as rapidly as ours. Ironically, for women who believe they have to drink milk to strengthen their bones, the high protein in dairy products binds with dairy's calcium, making this mineral less available for the body's needs (bones, nerve impulses, healthy blood pH).

Other dietary risk factors for osteoporosis are a high protein diet and high sodium intake. Eating a high-protein diet is one sure way to lose extra calcium and increase one's risk for osteoporosis. Women who eat less salt, protein, and sugar than is common in the standard American diet (all of which rob calcium from the body) have less need, if any, for calcium supplements.

For women in the higher-risk group for osteoporosis (see box), prevention can begin years before menopause. But if you have not yet taken precautions against

---

Risk Factors for Osteoporosis

No exercise

Smoking

No children

Drinking alcoholic beverages daily

Caffeine and soda (more than a total of five cups a day)

Excess fat in diet, especially animal fats, including dairy products

High-protein diet

High-sodium diet

Calcium supplements, especially without magnesium (Though a diet low in calcium is a risk factor, taking calcium in excess, as an isolated nutrient, is not as helpful and may even interfere with calcium bioavailability.)

Being underweight by more than 15 pounds

Being overweight by more than 25 pounds

Non-African-American ethnic group, especially Asian and Caucasian

Early age for starting menstruation

Early menopause

Past medical history of pathological fracture (without obvious cause or trauma)

Family history of osteoporosis

Family history of diabetes

Steroid drugs, especially with long-term use because of arthritis, asthma, or autoimmune disorders

Thyroid medication, especially with long-term use

---

bone thinning, it's still not too late. The truth is, for women who don't have a large number of risk factors (see box), the best prevention is exercise, whole food nutrition, and, when necessary, herbs to nourish the blood and bones and encourage healthy levels of postmenopausal hormones.

Please remember that it takes more than one risk factor to cause a multifactorial disease such as osteoporosis. Panic about having a few risk factors is not as helpful as changing what you can. When you have started to do that, you can relax about the few things you may not be able to change.

Herbal Medicine

In the following formulas, the diuretic action of dandelion leaf and root helps the kidneys excrete any excess calcium and avoid kidney stones, but never by removing it from bone. Dandelion leaf is also naturally rich in potassium, which we need when we take diuretics—yet another example of nature's inherent wisdom. This multipurpose herb is also a digestive bitter that helps rebalance normal stomach acid if you have been using an excess of calcium supplements.

Herbs rich in calcium and other minerals are best taken as a tea because the water assists in bioavailability. The next two combinations can also strengthen skin, nails, and hair in three or more months. If your mane becomes glossy and you run like the wind, just be careful where you start to sow those wild oats.

❧ ——————————WILD HORSES TONIC—————————— ❧

Extracts	Botanical Names	Actions
2 oz. wild oat herb	*Avena sativa*	Provides minerals; nourishes nerves, skin, hair
2 oz. horsetail herb	*Equisetum arvense*	Helps kidneys, elimination; provides minerals
1 oz. dandelion root, raw	*Taraxacum officinale*	Helps elimination, liver, digestion
1 oz. dandelion root, roasted	*Taraxacum officinale*	Adds minerals; for taste
1 oz. dandelion leaf	*Taraxacum officinale*	Reduces water retention, adds minerals
1 oz. nettle leaf	*Urtica dioica*	Nutritive; supports immune resistance
1 oz. yellow dock root	*Rumex crispus*	Stimulates liver; aids fat metabolism; adds iron
1 oz. alfalfa herb	*Medicago sativa*	Nutritive; relieves stiffness; provides gentle hormonal effects

Ten ounces will last thirty days. Combine these herbal extracts. Take 1 teaspoon twice a day (in the morning and evening) in 1 cup water, juice, or any herb tea.

——————————————WILD HORSES TEA——————————————

Dried Herbs	Botanical Names	Actions
3 oz. wild oat herb	*Avena sativa*	Provides minerals; nourishes nerves, skin, hair
2 oz. horsetail herb	*Equisetum arvense*	Helps kidneys, elimination; provides minerals
2 oz. dandelion root, raw	*Taraxacum officinale*	Helps elimination, liver, digestion
2 oz. dandelion root, roasted	*Taraxacum officinale*	Adds minerals; for taste
2 oz. dandelion leaf	*Taraxacum officinale*	Reduces water retention, adds minerals
2 oz. nettle leaf	*Urtica dioica*	Nutritive; supports immune resistance
1 oz. yellow dock root	*Rumex crispus*	Stimulates liver; aids fat metabolism; adds iron
1 oz. alfalfa herb	*Medicago sativa*	Nutritive; relieves stiffness; provides gentle hormonal effects

Fifteen ounces will last thirty days. Add 1/2 ounce of the mixture to 4 cups of boiling water in a teapot or container with a well-fitting lid. Let stand for twenty minutes before straining. Drink 1 cup hot or cold three times a day. Or if you prefer, sip tea all day or drink two large glasses twice a day—just be sure to drink 3 cups a day.

Nutrition

Wise Food Choices

- Calcium is widely available in nature, and most plants we eat have it in abundance. For nondairy sources of calcium that are easy on your heart, cholesterol, figure, and general health, eat dark green leafy vegetables, especially spinach, kale, dandelion greens, watercress, chard, and parsley. Fresh raw nuts and seeds such as almonds, sunflower seeds, pumpkin seeds, and particularly sesame seeds (including tahini) are also high in calcium.
- Vegetables can be steamed if the roughage causes digestive upsets. And do eat your spinach, even though it is getting bad press these days. Yes, spinach

contains oxalic acids that bind with calcium and decrease available iron, but it does different things when eaten raw, steamed, with other foods, or all by itself. Try preparing it as people in traditional cultures do: Drizzle a little lemon juice or a half-teaspoon of raw organic apple cider vinegar over combinations of steamed or raw spinach and other green leafy vegetables; the acidic pH of the lemon juice makes the minerals in the greens more easily digestible. Though spinach has some oxalic acid, which should be avoided by people who are sensitive to its negative effects on arthritis, it is so full of chlorophyll and other good nutrients that people call it the "Friend of the Elderly."

- Each week eat two servings of tofu, a high-protein soy food that is rich in calcium, instead of meat, fish, or eggs. Avoid brands with added preservatives. Fresh tofu is available at natural-food stores or Asian groceries.
- Avoid refined sugars, which rob the body of calcium and interfere with blood sugar balance, energy, mood, and hormonal and immune system stability.

Supplements

- If you choose to use calcium supplements, remember that vitamin D (not the synthetic one in milk) helps absorption. Natural vitamin D synthesis in your body occurs when sunshine is allowed to fall on your skin. This does not mean tanning salons or risking skin cancer at the beach. Taking a walk is a way to supplement vitamin D and get your cardiovascular house in order. Also, women need to balance calcium the way nature does, with the right ratio of magnesium. If you truly need supplements, don't bother with ones containing an aluminum-based antiacid or alkaline carrier because they interfere with the stomach acid needed to absorb calcium. Double the magnesium-to-calcium ratio in your supplementation. For example, if you take 1,200 milligrams of calcium, and the RDA (recommended daily allowance) of magnesium is 280 milligrams for women, take 560–600 milligrams of magnesium.
- Vitamin C, preferably from food sources as described in "Hot Flashes and Night Sweats"

In Addition

- Exercise. Women hate it or love it. If you love it already, you can skip this part. If you hate it, don't ever do it again. That's right! What you want to do instead is *move*. The general discussion on exercise earlier in this section provides suggestions on healthy ways to move. In traditional cultures where movement is not "exercise," but just part of using your body every day, women do not worry about broken hips or the price of gym shorts. Forget exercise. Discover how you like to move, and don't look back.

- Now is the time to gain in physical fitness and drop excess weight—if at all possible without self-judgment or getting depressed. Just start wherever you are.
- Avoid fluoride in toothpaste and water because it interferes with calcium absorption.
- Protect yourself from pollution—for example, by getting away to the country more often and by removing toxic chemicals from your home and yard.
- Check with your physician to see if your medications (antacids with aluminum, heparin, steroids for arthritis, thyroid hormones, anticonvulsants) can be switched or reduced to minimize their effects on bone loss.
- Limit alcohol, caffeine, and smoking.
- Reread the list of risk factors to see what else you can do.

Depression

The changes women undergo in the course of their lives have long seemed mysterious and were feared by men and women alike. Even at the turn of the twentieth century, some menopausal women were institutionalized for "involutional melancholia," a term for menopausal depression. Conventional medicine continues to focus on pathology even where menopause is concerned, viewing it as a "failure" of the ovaries to produce adequate estrogen and proposing surgical and pharmaceutical options to cure it. But menopausal women are not deficient. We are not failing. We may need supportive health advice but not automatic replacement of a hormone that the body was designed to lower at this time of life.

If you feel unable to cope with stress or your emotions seem out of control during menopause, the cause is likely to be changes in your hormonal balance, which is partly controlled by the adrenal glands. One job of the adrenal glands is to make adrenaline and other hormones that help us respond to stress. A related function is making small amounts of sex hormones. After menopause, the adrenal glands continue to make a little estrogen and other steroidal hormones, but mainly they take the androstenedione that our ovaries continue to produce and convert it into the hormone estrone, which has beneficial effects like those of estrogen. Therefore, taking care of your adrenals before and during menopause is a good way to ensure that you improve your changing tolerance to stress and depression. The herbs in the following formulas can help optimize adrenal health and also help you gain more natural control over your body's own balance of estrogen and its close relative, estrone.

After an initial period of unpredictability, you'll find that your response to stress improves as your body adjusts to its new hormonal balance. The process is similar to what happens after rearranging furniture: You are used to having it the old way and initially may bump into the furniture, but very soon you get used to the new pathways.

If you experience suicidal feelings during menopause, they are not necessarily a sign of severe mental disease, but rather of depression resulting from your changing hormonal balance. But by no means should you ignore these feelings: Seek the company of a trusted friend or the counsel of a mental health professional to uncover their causes. The process may well bring you to an important evaluation of your previous years of life, one in which you experience the "death" of what has gone before. As in the loss of someone close to you, you may need to work through your grief of that loss, moving through shock and grief to recovery. The butterfly is the Mexican spiritual symbol of the soul for this very good reason: The old life form must pass away before the new form takes flight in harmony and beauty. Allow yourself to cocoon and renew if that is what you need. Consider trying the following supportive tonics and other healing herbs. Pay attention to lifestyle changes, rather than short-circuiting the symptoms with mood-altering substances such as alcohol or even continued estrogen therapy, or overuse of Prozac or other antidepressant drugs. (Antidepressants can prevent suicidal mood swings with or without menopausal symptoms, but they are too commonly prescribed.)

Herbal Medicine

The following formulas use menopausal remedies with complementary properties to ease nagging aches and depression, such as black cohosh *(Cimicifuga racemosa),* wild yam root *(Dioscorea villosa),* and St. John's wort *(Hypericum perforatum)*. Many of these "nervines" (herbs benefiting the nerves) have an affinity for encouraging healthy reproductive function. Used together, damiana *(Turnera diffusa)* and black cohosh relax muscles, lessen pain, calm the nerves, and strengthen the body. This combined benefit often enables women to cope better with all the taxing changes of dealing with self-image and sexuality during menopause. For example, the long-term use of St. John's wort has been found to be successful in helping women come off antidepressants such as Valium. For an antidepressant effect, it should be used for minimum of eight weeks. To wean off Valium, this is best done under the supervision of a qualified and sympathetic care provider who is familiar with herbs and Valium. Black cohosh is contained in many standard European and American menopausal formulas because it helps normalize natural estrogen levels and reduce nervous tension. It has an affinity for decreasing joint pain and stabilizing mood swings; it also has the bonus effect of toning the lungs. The following combinations are recommended for depression, emotional vulnerability, and nervous tension. Think of them as all-natural fuel for the little engine that said, "I think I can, I think I can." Though neither extract nor tea is a delightful-tasting beverage, one or both will lighten your mood while strengthening your power. If you wish, add honey or other delicious herbs (peppermint, fennel, hibiscus) to taste. If you have blood sugar problems, don't use sugar or more than 1 teaspoon of honey per cup.

Extracts	Botanical Names	Actions
4 oz. black cohosh root	*Cimicifuga racemosa*	Adjusts low estrogen; relaxes nerves
4 oz. St. John's wort herb	*Hypericum perforatum*	Repairs nerve damage; acts as antidepressant
4 oz. Siberian ginseng root	*Eleutherococcus senticosus*	Improves response to stress
2 oz. lavender flower	*Lavandula officinalis*	Lifts spirits; is cleansing and soothing
1 oz. vervain herb	*Verbena officinalis*	Tones liver; balances mood, hormones
1 oz. licorice root	*Glycyrrhiza glabra*	Moistening; anti-inflammatory

Sixteen ounces will last thirty days or more depending on need. Combine the extracts. Take 1 teaspoon in 1 cup water, juice, or any herb tea three times a day. For immediate help in coping with difficult times in the short term, take 1/2 teaspoon every fifteen to twenty minutes, up to a total of 3 teaspoons (six doses) in two hours, plus the usual 3 teaspoons per day, as needed. These higher amounts can be continued for a week or two, especially if a crisis is also being handled through spot counseling or other appropriate help. If vervain is not available, replace it with 1/4 ounce of mugwort *(Artemisia vulgaris)*. If desired, replace licorice with wild yam *(Dioscorea villosa)*.

CENTERED IN PEACE

Dried Herbs	Botanical Names	Actions
1 oz. damiana herb	*Turnera diffusa*	Stimulates nerves and sluggish digestion
3 oz. raspberry leaf	*Rubus idaeus*	Calming, nutritive; provides minerals; tones womb
3 oz. St. John's wort herb	*Hypericum perforatum*	Antidepressant; improves resistance
3 oz. lemon balm leaf	*Melissa officinalis*	For taste; improves digestion, mood
1 oz. borage flower	*Borago officinalis*	Cooling, nutritive
1/2 oz. motherwort herb	*Leonurus cardiaca*	Lessens hot flashes; strengthens heart
1/4 oz. calendula flower	*Calendula officinalis*	Tones liver, lymph, skin; anti-inflammatory
1/4 oz. rose petals	*Rosa* species	Tonic, astringent; for beauty

Fifteen ounces will last thirty days. Combine 1/2 ounce of the mixture with 3 1/2 cups of boiling water in a teapot or container with a well-fitting lid. Let stand for fifteen minutes before straining. Drink 1 cup hot or cold three times a day. One teapot as strong as you like can be used as often as needed. Or, if you prefer, sip tea all day or drink two large glasses twice a day, making sure you drink 3 cups a day. Take eight weeks or more for lasting benefits. If lemon balm or borage flowers are unavailable, replace with lemon verbena *(Lippia citriodora)*.

Nutrition

Wise Food Choices

- To improve liver metabolism, mood, and digestion, eat bitter, leafy vegetables like radicchio, endive, young dandelion greens, and kale. Also try edible flowers in salads, especially those in yellow-orange and blue-purple colors (these provide health-giving pigments, beta-carotene, and other nutrients), such as spicy nasturtiums and sweet violets.
- Avoid alcohol (though it may feel good at first, it is a nerve depressant; it also interacts with estrogen activity and can damage the liver).
- Avoid caffeine, chocolate (even though there is an adrenaline rush, it hurts the nerves and eventually worsens the adrenal stress response).

Supplements

- Evening primrose oil, borage, or flax seed, as directed on labels

Dysmenorrhea and Other Common Causes of Reproductive System Pain

Dysmenorrhea is a catch-all word meaning "painful or difficult menstrual bleeding." It can include cramps, painful arthritic inflammation, migraines, and pelvic pressure, perhaps with bloating or alternating diarrhea and constipation. Women in menopause often describe the pain as a dragging sensation. This achiness may come with a feeling that the contents of the pelvis are being pulled downward. These symptoms involve the reproductive and the nervous systems, so the herbs you use must help both. Used in conjunction with moderate exercise, a good diet, and abundant rest, the herbal remedies suggested below promote circulation, strengthen nerves, eliminate congestion, and bring better tone to the ligaments.

Sometimes a woman's pain threshold shifts around this time of the month and during the perimenopausal period. Because pain of any kind is an important message, the combinations in this section are designed so they will not suppress symptoms, but they are strong enough to take the edge off pain and provide some emergency relief. They can be used once or twice as needed for minor symptoms or for one to three months for more longstanding conditions. It takes at least ninety days for natural remedies to make significant improvements in chronic conditions. If symptoms don't feel "minor" to you, always know that a caring licensed health-care practitioner can rule out problems requiring more immediate attention.

Herbal Medicine

❦————————————— HERBAL 911————————————— ❦

Extracts	Botanical Names	Actions
4 oz. passion flower herb	*Passiflora incarnata*	Pain relieving, emotionally calming
4 oz. cramp bark	*Viburnum opulus*	Relaxes muscle spasms; relieves pain from tension
2 oz. valerian root	*Valeriana officinalis*	Sedates; relieves spasms; induces sleepiness

Ten ounces will last thirty days. Combine these herbal extracts. For pain relief *right now*, start with 10 drops every five minutes for twenty minutes. If that doesn't help, take 1/2 ounce diluted in 1/2 cup water, and sip over the next twenty minutes. Repeat as needed.

If you experience chronic dull or aching pain before, after, or during bleeding, take 1/2 teaspoon in water three times every day for three weeks before the next period and during bleeding if needed. If your cycle is erratic, so that "three weeks before" is impossible to predict, you can safely use the mixture all through the month and during bleeding.

If pain is caused by a diagnosed condition of uterine prolapse or blockage, add 2 ounces of the tissue tonic, blue cohosh *(Caulophyllum thalictroides)*. This can help you heal, but you may need to do more than take the tissue tonics and connective tissue remedies. Exercise, chiropractic or osteopathic adjustments, and acupuncture may help here. If severe pain isn't lessened at all within two hours, call for more specific advice from your nearest health-care provider. For chronic lower back pain during or after menopause, try this tonic tea.

❦————————————— I FEEL FREE TEA ————————————— ❦

Dried Herbs	Botanical Names	Actions
4 oz. passion flower herb	*Passiflora incarnata*	Pain relieving, emotionally calming
3 oz. black haw root bark	*Viburnum prunifolium*	Relaxes ovarian, uterine muscle spasms
2 oz. sage leaf	*Salvia officinalis*	Supports hormonal balance, digestion; for taste
1/2 oz. ginger root	*Zingiber officinale*	Improves circulation, metabolism; for taste

Fifteen ounces will last about thirty days. Combine 1/3 ounce of the mixture with 3 cups of boiling water in a teapot or container with a well-fitting lid. Let stand for fifteen minutes before straining. Drink 2 cups hot or cold as needed.

Painful intercourse caused by dysmenorrhea, fibroids, or loss of lubrication in the vaginal canal is also associated with menopause. Though sex helps all these conditions, it is hard to have good sex when it doesn't feel good. Many herbs are known to help women's enjoyment of sexuality by healing, toning, and calming inflamed vaginal tissue, lubricating thin walls, or relaxing taut muscles. For example, wound-healing herbs such as yarrow *(Achillea millefolium)* and calendula *(Calendula officinalis)* are toning and anti-inflammatory when used directly on vaginal tissues. They are particularly beneficial if pain is caused by dryness, infection, or irritation. The following herb formulas relieve pain while healing from the inside out; also see the recommendations in "Vaginal Thinning and Dryness."

Taken internally in tea form or as extracts, many of these same herbs are also digestive bitters. This is nature's way of feeding two birds with one morsel: hormonal and digestive changes are treated together. From the inside of the body, herbs can help relieve pelvic congestion, sluggish bowels, bloating, intestinal gas, and even heavy menstrual bleeding. Other digestive herbs with helpful properties for improving the integrity of the vaginal walls and uterine muscle during menopause are sage *(Salvia officinalis)*, licorice *(Glycyrrhiza glabra)*, and chamomile *(Matricaria recutita)*.

Different types of pain respond to different herbs. Many common types of pain related to menopause can respond to the following two combinations. These remedies work on hormonal balance, sensory nerve endings, and adrenal stress. They also improve pelvic congestion and satisfactory elimination by activating the liver rather than stimulating the wall of the colon. This makes them milder, safer, and more comfortable to use than fast-acting herbal laxatives such as senna. *Cascara sagrada,* senna pods, and other strong anthraquinone-containing herbs are still useful in a pinch for constipation, but they only work on a symptomatic level and can be harsh on the body. The digestive bitter tonics used here are better for balancing sluggish or congested bowels in conjunction with bloating, gas, or even some alternating looseness of stools. If there's nothing wrong with the digestive tract, these herbs are mild enough not to overstimulate elimination. The combination will still offer its pain-lessening and nourishing qualities.

(In Greek, *nepenthe* means "herb that soothes away sorrow.")

Extracts	Botanical Names	Actions
4 oz. passion flower herb	*Passiflora incarnata*	Pain relieving, emotionally calming
2 oz. licorice root	*Glycyrrhiza glabra*	Anti-inflammatory; moistening
2 oz. chamomile flower	*Matricaria recutita*	Calming to nerves, digestion; reduces bloating
1 oz. black cohosh root	*Cimicifuga racemosa*	Balances hormones; calms; anti-inflammatory
1 oz. wild yam root	*Dioscorea villosa*	Supports hormonal balance; anti-inflammatory

Ten ounces will last thirty days. Combine these herbal extracts. Take 1 teaspoon in 1 cup water, juice, or any herb tea in the morning and evening. If desired, replace licorice with skullcap *(Scutellaria* species*)*.

Dried Herbs	Botanical Names	Actions
5 oz. passion flower herb	*Passiflora incarnata*	Pain relieving, emotionally calming
3 oz. sage leaf	*Salvia officinalis*	Supports hormonal balance, digestion; for taste
3 oz. skullcap herb	*Scutellaria laterifolia*	Nourishes; soothes nervous tension
2 oz. chamomile flower	*Matricaria recutita*	Calming to nerves, digestion; reduces bloating
1 oz. dong quai root	*Angelica sinensis*	Increases low estrogen; builds immune reserves
1 oz. cinnamon bark	*Cinnamomum* species	Warms; tones; astringent

Fifteen ounces will last thirty days. Combine 1/2 ounce of the mixture with 4 cups boiling water in a teapot or container with a well-fitting lid. Let stand for fifteen minutes before straining. Drink 1 cup hot or cold two to four times a day, or if you prefer, sip tea all day. If you are allergic to the daisy family, especially chrysanthemums, replace the chamomile with an extra 1/2 ounce of cinnamon and 1 1/2 ounces of linden *(Tilia* species*)*.

If you need to sleep to give your body a chance to escape constant or chronic pain, use the following herb as a last resort for quick symptom relief:

Extract	Botanical Name	Actions
1 oz. valerian root	*Valeriana officinalis*	Pain relieving; sedates; relaxes muscle tension

Dilute 10 to 15 drops of this pungent root in water, juice, or herb tea and take every ten to fifteen minutes until pain is gone. This usually occurs in two to three doses; don't take more than ten doses in any two-hour period. By that point, sleep will be on the horizon anyway. A tea of the root, 1/2 ounce to a pint of water, is also effective though it doesn't taste good and smells peculiar; drink a teacup at a time as needed. Nonalcohol extracts with glycerin are available in many stores and taste better but are slightly less effective.

Yet another cause of pain is the menstrual migraine. This form of headache also may flare up in menopause and is aggravated by excess estrogen, caffeine, and other factors. Prevention is the best remedy for these headaches whether they are related to the menstrual cycle or changing estrogen levels in menopause. Prevention includes eating regularly to stabilize blood sugar, releasing tension before it builds up, and taking herbs to ease premenstrual or menopausal irritability. When it is too late for prevention, try one or more of the following three remedies to make an immediate difference. There are three choices because each will not work for every woman, and you may need to experiment to get the relief you need.

❧ ————— NUMB SKULL COMPOUND ————— ❧

Extracts	Botanical Names	Actions
2 oz. skullcap herb	*Scutellaria laterifolia*	Relaxes tension, anxiety; nourishes nerves
2 oz. lavender flower	*Lavandula officinalis*	Cleanses; relaxes; lifts spirits
2 oz. motherwort herb	*Leonurus cardiaca*	Lowers tension, high blood pressure

Six ounces will last a long time without refrigeration; keep on hand for occasional headaches. Combine these herbal extracts. Take 1 to 3 teaspoons in 1 cup water, juice, or any herb tea up to ten times a day if needed. At maximum dose, that's 30 teaspoons or just over 4 ounces in a day, so be sure to drink plain water and other fluids, eat small meals, and rest. If your headache requires that much tincture, avoid driving; instead, stay home or take a stress-relieving walk.

Extracts	Botanical Names	Actions
4 oz. skullcap herb	*Scutellaria laterifolia*	Reduces pressure, tension
2 oz. rosemary flower, leaf	*Rosmarinus officinalis*	Relaxes blood vessels
2 oz. linden flower	*Tilia* species	Reduces high blood pressure; calms; moistens
1 oz. sage leaf	*Salvia officinalis*	Supports hormonal balance; tonic, astringent
1 oz. passion flower herb	*Passiflora incarnata*	Reduces physical, emotional pain

Ten ounces stored in a closed container away from direct heat and light will last up to a year without refrigeration. Combine 1/2 ounce of the mixture with 3 cups of boiling water in a teapot or container with a well-fitting lid. Let stand for five to fifteen minutes before straining. Drink 2 cups hot or cold, as needed.

If you experience menstrual migraines, which are caused by blood vessel spasms, prevention is even more necessary than for tension headaches. The best herbal remedies for this type of headache do not get rid of a migraine once you have it; rather, they build up your resistance to future headaches. The main extract, feverfew *(Chrysanthemum parthenium),* must be made from the fresh flowering herb because dried tea has far less of an effect. Most companies know this; check the label of any store-bought extract to be sure it is from fresh plant material. Some women report that freeze-dried capsules work; others report they do not. When you feel like closing the door, disconnecting the phone, or heading for the hills, do that and take a cup of the following remedy.

Extracts	Botanical Names	Actions
3 oz. fresh feverfew herb	*Chrysanthemum parthenium*	Stabilizes blood vessels to brain
2 oz. chasteberry seed	*Vitex agnus-castus*	Stabilizes hormones
1 oz. lavender flower	*Lavandula officinalis*	Cleanses; relaxes; uplifts
2 oz. sage leaf	*Salvia officinalis*	Tonic, astringent; supports hormonal balance

Take 1 teaspoon diluted in a cup of liquid every morning; to mask its odd taste, try it in diluted fruit juice or herb tea (try "Floral Calm," above). Take an extra dose if you feel a migraine sneaking up on you.

When all is said and done, pain is sometimes not just physical or just emotional. When you know the cause of severe pain, but it has not responded to the gentle methods described above, it is not wrong or weak to suppress it. Allowing yourself escape routes in severe distress can allow your body's resources to mobilize for deep healing. A recent study shows that symptom-suppressing pain medication prescribed immediately after an operation can allow more rapid healing. The use of nature's painkillers can also contribute to healing in this way.

When physical or emotional pain is severe, take up to 1 ounce of passion flower tincture diluted in one 8-ounce cup of water or herb tea. If pain in your lower back or abdomen is causing insomnia, try massaging the affected area with the aromatherapy blend noted under "In Addition." Or take a lavender bath or even a warm shower that ends with a lukewarm or cool rinse. Then return to bed with a cup of sleep-inducing herb tea. This can be the "Good Night" formula included in "Changes in the Nervous System" in Chapter 4 or a single herb, from mild chamomile to medium-strong motherwort (very bitter tasting) to the stronger valerian (strong tasting). Of these, only the chamomile tastes good as a tea to most women, so other useful forms are capsules (which may take up to an hour and a half to take effect) or glycerin tinctures, which have no alcohol. Alcohol-based tinctures work as well, but if you need to avoid alcohol (even a small amount of alcohol can trigger migraines in some women), do not use them. See "Herbal Preparations," at the end of this book, for more information.

The amount of alcohol in herbal extracts is relatively little when taken as directed, so if a small quantity of alcohol is not a problem for you, you can, of course, use alcohol-based tinctures. It is the herb, not the alcohol, that is having the effect, so you are not really using the tincture as a stiff snort, as some skeptics might scoff. If one is in great pain, it will not help to sip 1 to 3 teaspoons of Scotch diluted in a cup of water before bed. However, this dose or less of the herb extracts can work wonders. This way of using herbs is not repeated long term, but it does work well for short-term symptom management of pain or insomnia.

The purpose of using these particular pain-lessening herb formulas is not to suppress each symptom but to improve the quality of life *in the moment* while we are still working on the causes of our discomfort. Returning to sleep in itself allows deeper self-healing, even if the sleep is achieved some nights with repeated doses of valerian. Remember, we are still discussing strong plant preparations, not habit-forming pharmaceutical drugs.

Nutrition

Wise Food Choices

- Avoid animal fats, including dairy and goat cheese, because they form prostaglandins, a large group of powerful hormonelike compounds that act locally on blood vessels, pain receptors, and a wide range of life processes.

Prostaglandins from animal protein and fat lower the pain threshold, worsening painful cramping. (One type of prostaglandins worsens pain and inflammation, while other prostglandins have totally opposite and even unrelated effects.)

- Drink plain water for all kinds of headaches.
- Eat a piece of fruit or a small meal to alleviate stress headaches or raise low blood sugar, which may itself cause headaches or worsen stress response.
- If you have painful periods with heavy flow and clotting, eat more carrots; drink 8 ounces of carrot juice a day for ten days before each cycle to lessen clotting.

In Addition

- To help relieve headaches, close your eyes for fifteen minutes.
- For headaches, especially when you are tired, massage just five or ten drops of essential oil of lavender and/or rosemary into the temples and back of neck.
- For stress, if you have time, add 5 to 10 drops of lavender or chamomile essential oil to a relaxing bath.
- Aromatherapy blend for pain:

    1 oz. almond, sesame, or olive oil
    25 drops essential oil of ginger
    15 drops essential oil of juniper
    10 drops essential oil of clary sage

Combine the essential oils with almond, sesame, or olive oil. Massage into painful lower back, thighs, and buttocks and down backs of legs. Repeat as often as needed. Use externally only. If skin sensitivity develops, discontinue use and wash with cool water and a mild soap; pat dry.

Hot Flashes and Night Sweats

In Great Britain and Australia, hot flashes are known as "flushing." For the longest time, I thought it was their accent, but they really do say, "Poor dear, she's having a hot flush." For many women, hot flashes are no joke. They can be the most debilitating symptom of menopause, though they can improve or even disappear through natural means. A hot flash is a sudden sensation of heat from blood vessels near the skin, sometimes with profuse sweating and sometimes preceded by chills. A hot flash starts in the chest and rises up the neck and face, and though it happens from head to toe, it is felt most in the upper body. Hot flashes that occur at night, especially with more perspiration, are called "night sweats." Generally, women who build up their health can soften the negative symptoms of hot flashes, some reporting that hot flashes become so minor that they are felt as pleasurable little waves.

When a hot flash occurs, what is happening in your body? The hot flash begins in the hypothalamus, a part of the brain. Among other things, the hypothalamus controls body temperature and, through feedback from the body, it regulates estrogen levels. When estrogen starts to drop in an uneven stop-and-start style, as frequently happens during menopause, the hypothalamus sends a chemical messenger—gonadotropin-releasing hormone, or GNRH—to the pituitary gland. The GNRH tells the pituitary to send follicle-stimulating hormone (FSH) to the ovaries; in turn, FSH politely requests the ovaries to hurry up with some estrogen by stimulating an egg follicle to develop with its usual yield of ovarian estrogen. The ovaries will or won't respond to this stimulus, depending on their ability to do so. Around menopause the ovaries may not have enough viable eggs left in the ovaries.

If an egg follicle develops under the influence of FSH, the estrogen it produces builds up to a certain level. Then this higher level of estrogen gives feedback to the brain to stop sending out FSH. If there is no viable egg left to develop, there is no ovulation, so there is no high buildup of estrogen, so there is no feedback to the brain. The result? The pituitary in the brain causes FSH to soar, trying to meet the usual goal of stimulating increased estrogen by repeating itself more loudly.

So now what? If the ovary cannot comply with the usual orders from the brain, the body responds to low estrogen by trying to storm the hypothalamus with adrenaline to get it moving. This tempest in a teapot affects the hypothalamus's temperature-control center, resetting the body's thermostat control for heat to reach a higher temperature, as if you were turning up the thermostat on your home's heating system. During a hot flash, you may actually feel a little chill before your body temperature feels hot-hot-hot in comparison to the new setting. The heart rate responds to the adrenaline's effect on the hypothalamus by speeding up a little or a lot, depending on the woman or the strength of each particular hot flash. The sensation starts in the chest and spreads up to the neck, face, and head. Then the skin gets involved. All the blood vessels, from the heart to the skin, dilate, allowing the body to cool by evaporation and bringing the temperature down to the new temperature set by the hypothalamus.

Hot flashes are affected by stress, any form of heat (from the weather outside to a lover's body in bed), and "vasodilators," substances that dilate the blood vessels: hot coffee, chili, and alcohol. Though nicotine causes blood vessels to contract, smoking also worsens hot flashes. Even menopause itself makes the blood vessels more vulnerable to temperature signals. Our blood vessels are more sensitive to drops and surges in estrogen and other hormones at this time. The body's feedback system notices all this flurry and checks to see why the temperature control was reset. After a while, your body gets tired of playing this exciting game, and figures out how to be at peace with its lower levels of estrogen. The feedback system has tried all its usual controls and finally sees that this is no temporary glitch. It is time for a new state of hormone balance. It is time for a Change.

Because women's blood vessels become more sensitive to sharp drops and floods of chemicals including hormones during the Change, the objective of taking certain herbs at this time is twofold: to stabilize blood vessel sensitivity to changing hormone levels, and to slow down or smooth the overall drop in estrogen from the ovaries. Some of these herbs do this by supporting the adrenal function. Our adrenals provide a little estrogen as a hormonal cushion. Adrenal tonic herbs, called "adaptogens," help our adrenal glands help us to *adapt* to current levels of stress. Examples are Siberian ginseng *(Eleutherococcus senticosus)*, borage *(Borago officinalis)*, ginseng *(Panax ginseng)*, and nettle *(Urtica dioica)*.

Nervines are another category of herbs that do more than simply suppress hot flashes: They help the body handle stress by providing relaxation, stimulation, or pain relief. They can mitigate hot flashes because, as every woman knows from experience and recent research has shown, the endocrine (hormone) and nervous systems are not two separate systems—each improves or worsens depending on the health or strain on the other. Nourishing herbs like motherwort *(Leonurus cardiaca)* that calm frazzled nerve endings can help make hot flashes disappear or at least be more comfortable (in severe cases, more tolerable).

One particular herb or another in this section may relieve hot flashes time and again for some women. But for severe or stubborn hot flashes, more women find better results from combinations of herbs that support the liver's natural function of metabolizing circulating hormones and the estrogen still made in our bodies. Wisely combined formulas also optimize the function of all types of estrogen, from ovaries, adrenal glands, and even fat cells. Hormonal tonics such as licorice *(Glycyrrhiza glabra)* can do double-duty by optimizing liver function and acting on the adrenal glands as a nourishing tonic.

Night sweats and palpitations (feeling your heart pound) can be addressed with herbal cardiovascular tonics, nervine relaxants, and hormonal balancers such as dong quai *(Angelica sinensis)*, motherwort *(Leonurus cardiaca)*, linden *(Tilia platyphylla/T. europea)*, and yarrow *(Achillea millefolium)*. These four plants, used singly or in any combination, stabilize the sensitivity of blood vessels to ebbs and flows in estrogen. Each of these has its own particular benefit, and no one needs them all, so choose the most appropriate one (for descriptions of the herbs, see the "Materia Medica" at the end of the book). The following two formulas strengthen and tone the blood vessels and, through the addition of hormone balancers such as chasteberry *(Vitex agnus-castus)*, normalize your system's changing amounts of estrogen.

Herbal Medicine

ENGINE COOLER

Extracts	Botanical Names	Actions
3 oz. chasteberry seed	*Vitex agnus-castus*	Stabilizes drops and surges in hormones
2 oz. motherwort herb	*Leonurus cardiaca*	Cools symptoms; calms heart palpitations
2 oz. hawthorn flower, leaf, berry	*Crataegus* species	Protects heart; strengthens blood vessels
2 oz. yarrow flower	*Achillea millefolium*	Cools temperature; stimulates liver
1 oz. dong quai root	*Angelica sinensis*	Supports estrogen balance; builds healthy blood

Ten ounces will last thirty days. Combine these herbal extracts. Every ten minutes take one dropper or 1/4 teaspoon diluted in 1/4 cup of room-temperature water. This remedy usually works in two to three doses, but the effect won't last long unless you take it consistently. For more permanent improvement, take 1 teaspoon three times a day for two weeks; then take a few days off and repeat for another two weeks. After that, repeat as needed. "Engine Cooler" combines well with the tea described below. The "cucumber" in the tea is really borage, a flowering edible plant whose peeled stalk smells and tastes a little like cucumbers. The overall effect of this tea is stabilizing, soothing, and moistening.

COOL AS A CUCUMBER TEA

Dried Herbs	Botanical Names	Actions
1 oz. motherwort herb	*Leonurus cardiaca*	Cools hot flashes; lessens sweating
2 oz. linden flower	*Tilia* species	Relaxes nerves; lowers high blood pressure
1 oz. chamomile flower	*Matricaria recutita*	Soothes stomach, nerves
4 oz. skullcap herb	*Scutellaria laterifolia*	Eases tension; nourishes frazzled nerves
3 oz. borage flowers, stems, and leaves	*Borago officinalis*	Moistens; nutritive tonic
2 oz. marshmallow root	*Althaea officinalis*	Moistens; helps water balance
2 oz. hibiscus flower	*Hibiscus sabdariffa*	Cooling; for taste

Fifteen ounces will last thirty days. Combine 1 ounce of the mixture with 4 cups of boiling water in a teapot or container with a well-fitting lid. Let stand for fifteen minutes; then strain the tea and store it in a closed container. Allow to cool; drink at room temperature—not hot and not icy cold. During daytime hot flashes, drink 1 cup as often as needed. Or, if you prefer, sip this amount of tea all day or drink two large glasses twice a day—just be sure you drink it all sometime each day. The tea is also good for sipping while you are drying off from a cool bath or shower. Drink 1/2 to 3 cups as needed after night sweats before you return to a fresh, dry bed, but remember to empty the bladder before going to sleep.

Hops and valerian are stronger sleep-inducing herb teas or tinctures than the combinations above and taste correspondingly stronger. Either or both may replace linden and skullcap in the formula above at those times when the mind needs to turn off so the body can sleep deeply. For fewer hot flashes and sounder sleep, try 1 to 2 cups of the herbal formula earlier during the evening to help the body wind down before bedtime. Remember to empty the bladder the last thing before bed so you aren't awakened from a sound sleep for a midnight trip to the bathroom.

Nutrition

Wise Food Choices

- Choose foods that are high in vitamin C. Among the many options are citrus fruits; rosehip jam (although vitamin C is lost in cooking except in some high-quality brands, natural fruit pectins and bioflavonoids offer fiber and other benefits to vessel tone); fresh, raw, green, sweet bell peppers; fresh, raw broccoli (raw broccoli is high in C; lightly steamed or stir-fried is okay).
- Avoid cayenne pepper and other hot spices. Cayenne may seem like a good food source of vitamin C, but stimulating spices aggravate hot flashes, causing blood vessels at the skin's surface to open up and evaporate the heat; the resulting perspiration cools down the body.
- Avoid caffeine (including soft drinks, chocolate, and aspirin containing caffeine) and alcohol.
- Great alternatives to the supplements listed below are home-sprouted seeds and nuts, rich in essential fatty acids, proteins, and enzymes, and easy for menopausal women to assimilate.
- Also highly recommended are foods rich in natural plant estrogens (phytoestrogens) that augment our own estrogen, such as soy flour, red clover sprouts, and flax seeds. For more information about these foods, see "Herbs and Nutrition in Menopause" earlier in this chapter.

Supplements

- Some women find that 600 to 800 I.U. (international units) of vitamin E taken daily is useful for hot flashes. For better metabolization of dosages higher than 600 I.U., you can add 1 to 3 grams of vitamin C (1,000 to 3,000 milligrams) and divide the mixture into three equal doses. For example, in the morning, at midday, and in the evening, you would take 200 I.U. of vitamin E with 1 gram of C. After a week you should be able to reduce your intake of vitamin E to 400 I.U. daily. But please know that more is *not* better! It is best not to take more than 1,200 I.U. daily in long-term use. The conservative recommended limit is 100 I.U. daily if you have diabetes, hypertension, or a rheumatic heart condition.
- Evening primrose oil in capsules is also effective for hot flashes. Most research suggests the minimum dose in a range of 6 to 10 capsules a day. Though evening primrose oil is expensive, it may be effective in as quickly as three to six weeks, so you may find it to be an affordable option. Taking less or taking it sporadically seems to have little or no effect in some women, though for others even 2 to 4 capsules a day may help.

Single herbs make fine dietary supplements for managing the symptom of hot flashes or night sweats.

- Motherwort metabolizes fats and hormones, filters blood, and improves immunity. It is specifically helpful for heart palpitations as well as menopausal hot flashes and healthy liver function, so it may be useful in any formula taken by a woman with cardiovascular concerns. Dosage of store-bought extract ranges from 1 dropper to 1 teaspoon every ten to twenty minutes as needed and/or three times a day for prevention.
- Ginseng (*Panax ginseng*, also called Asian, Chinese, Korean, or Manchurian ginseng) taken for six weeks and longer works well too, although it may not work equally well in all women. (While other types of ginseng may not work as well in the short term for hot flashes, they are described in the "Materia Medica"—see "American ginseng" and "Siberian ginseng.") Some traditional Chinese medical practitioners say that menopausal women should never take ginseng. Nevertheless, numerous women have told me of the benefits it gave them, and there is research to support both views. Women who seem to react badly to ginseng are, to begin with, tired but high-strung, tense, and wound up. Women who do well with a little ginseng tend to feel, before taking the herb, emptied out, weakened in every body system, and slow to get going. The use of ginseng is certainly easier on a woman than HRT. The temporary "ginseng headache" that helps a person determine that this powerful herb may not be right for her is not as difficult a side effect to clear up as the cancer risk associated with replacement hormones.

- Licorice is a rich, affordable source of phytoestrogens. Although it should be used with some caution, moderate amounts or the conservative dosages suggested in this book are going to be helpful to most women going through the Change. An explanation of precautions is found in "Irregular Cycles," following, and in the full description of licorice in the "Materia Medica." Formulas including this herb also indicate substitutes.
- Natural sources of phytoestrogens commonly available in herb shops or natural-food stores require a different kind of caution. Sarsaparilla is often adulterated (mixed with other herb substitutes), so check with the herb seller to make sure you are buying pure Jamaican sarsaparilla, *Smilax ornata* or a related *Smilax* species. Real sarsaparilla has little fragrance; the more delicious the smell, the more likely it is to be a different plant confusingly called sarsaparilla. Because of rampant overharvesting, do not purchase the endangered wild American ginseng *(Panax quinquefolius)*. Please use only cultivated roots, grown and harvested with ecological sensitivity.

In Addition

- If you are having sudden hot flashes, wear light layers of cotton clothing. During a hot flash, try leaving the room for a change of scene or loosening your collar.
- Because hot flashes and sweating often worsen at night, you may want to open windows before bedtime if it is safe and practical to do so.
- Night sweats can drench a bed, so invest in two sets of cotton or linen bedding, and keep the extra set and other comfortable bedding at hand. Women report that imagining that day's problems confined to the pile of damp sheets wadded on the floor, destined for tomorrow's laundry, is helpful to them. If you feel the need to shower, wash in warm water and end with cooler water. Cooling off after a warm shower sends blood from peripheral vessels back to the interior of the body, indirectly resulting in a neuronal message directing your body to get drowsy. Keep a thermos or other container of "Good Night Tea" (see Chapter 4, "Postmenopause") in a convenient place nearby to further help you get back to sleep.

Though all this may seem like an undue amount of nighttime activity when you are fatigued, these steps help you focus your attention on returning to a comfortable bed for a few more hours of real sleep, instead of tossing about in a damp bed and drinking ever-stronger sleep-inducing herbs without the desired effect. I do not normally recommend strong "knock-out" herbs to get to sleep or return to sleep. Rather, women do well when they accept that there may be a temporary break in sleep. Many report that an attitude of calm acceptance allows the disturbance to be minimized in the mind, and thus minimized in fact.

Irregular Cycles

First you have a late period. Then you have two in just six weeks. You haven't bled in six months and think, "Hey, that was easy!" but the next month there's a scarlet stain on your white sheets. When your biological clock starts winding down, your cycle becomes irregular and your emotions may well become unpredictable.

The best way you can cope is to really take care of yourself. Deeply focus on stabilizing your body: Prolong your naturally occurring estrogen levels, build your health, look beyond symptoms that come and go, nourish each of the body systems affected by the Change. Focus your inner being by drawing more love to yourself in your personal, social, and spiritual relationships. Tall order? Your energy and your spirit are limitless.

And nature offers some kind assistance. One or more of the hormonal normalizers found in every habitat on Earth, such as the North American black cohosh, support a grace-filled Change, as does chasteberry *(Vitex agnus-castus)*, a Mediterranean seed in human use as a hormonal tonic for more than three thousand years.

China introduced dong quai *(Angelica sinensis)* root to the West, but my Euro-American tradition favors the use of chasteberry. In Europe, older herbal practitioners with whom I did my internship swore they could not treat menopause safely and effectively without this pungent seed. It may be that during other decades in the twentieth century, herbal alternatives such as American ginseng, red clover, and the cohoshes were not as fresh or high quality as chasteberry. Chinese herbs used for women in menopause, such as dong quai, bupleurum *(Bupleurum Chinense)*, and other companion herbs, were relatively unknown to Euro-American herbal traditions until recent years. False unicorn root *(Chamaelirium luteum)*, which was a standard American remedy, is endangered in the wild, and so ethical herbal practitioners will not use it unless they personally collect it where it is locally abundant, even though it is still recommended in mass-produced herb books and formulas. Nature is generous in giving us several equally good herbs in the hormone-balancing category, so if we do not wish to destroy the plants we know and love, let us be equally generous in returning a little of our time to nature.

Herbal Medicine

Compared to the "Ancient Clock, Perfect Timing" formulas in Chapter 1, the following two formulas and tea are more nourishing for women in menopause. For the quickest results, "Lunar Nectar" works with the power of the moon's pull on gravity to establish a regular menses, even if it is not twenty-eight days. If your cycles have been erratic for longer than six months, use the "Womb Rhythm" formula or tea instead.

Extracts	Botanical Names	Actions
4 oz. chasteberry seed	*Vitex agnus-castus*	Regulates pituitary control of hormones
2 oz. black cohosh root	*Cimicifuga racemosa*	Reduces tension; helps balance estrogen
2 oz. nettle leaf	*Urtica dioica*	Nutritive; supports liver, kidney function
2 oz. rosehips	*Rosa canina*	Nutritive; provides bioflavonoids; cooling
1 oz. motherwort herb	*Leonurus cardiaca*	Calms, strengthens heart
1 oz. dong quai root	*Angelica sinensis*	Moistens; builds blood, low estrogen levels

Twelve ounces will last thirty days. Combine these herbal extracts. Take 1 teaspoon in 1 cup water, juice, or any herb tea three times a day (morning, afternoon (3 to 5 P.M.) and after dinner. Though it may bring improvement in the first month, take for a minimum of three months for better results.

Extracts	Botanical Names	Actions
2 oz. fresh shepherd's purse herb	*Capsella bursa-pastoris*	Stops or slows excess bleeding
2 oz. lady's mantle leaf	*Alchemilla vulgaris*	Protects reproductive tissue
1 oz. blue cohosh root	*Caulophyllum thalictroides*	Balances hormones; astringent
1 oz. black cohosh root	*Cimicifuga racemosa*	Balances hormones; relaxes
1 oz. chasteberry seed	*Vitex agnus-castus*	Lowers excess estrogen

Seven ounces will last approximately a week; this amount lasts three days or so if the higher dose is needed for short-term results. Combine these extracts; take 1 to 3 teaspoons every two hours until bleeding stops or slows down. For chronic problems with spotting between cycles, flooding, and fibroids, take 1 teaspoon three times a day for a minimum of three months (15 ounces per month).

Dried Herbs	Botanical Names	Actions
4 oz. chasteberry seed	*Vitex agnus-castus*	Lessens excess estrogen
3 oz. sage leaf	*Salvia officinalis*	Balances hormones; astringent
3 oz. partridge berry herb	*Mitchella repens*	Lessens excess bleeding; tones
3 oz. lady's mantle herb	*Alchemilla vulgaris*	Protects reproductive tissues
1 oz. yellow dock root	*Rumex crispus*	Stimulates liver; helps iron assimilation
1 oz. cinnamon bark	*Cinnamonum zeylanicum*	For taste; soothes; lessens bleeding

Fifteen ounces will last thirty days. Add 1 ounce of the mixture to 4 cups of boiling water in a teapot or container with a well-fitting lid. Let stand for fifteen minutes before straining. Drink 1 cup hot or cold, three to four times a day. Or, if you prefer, sip tea all day or drink two large glasses twice a day, but be sure you drink 3 or 4 cups of tea in a day.

Some women find that they would like to switch to a better-tasting tea after using this mixture for a month or two. This is perfectly normal and may occur because their taste buds change as their bodies respond. Here is an alternative tea that you can switch to at any time.

Dried Herbs	Botanical Names	Actions
4 oz. chasteberry seed	*Vitex agnus-castus*	Tones reproductive tissues
2 1/2 oz. wild oats herb	*Avena sativa*	Relaxes nerves; tones skin, hair
2 1/2 oz. raspberry leaf	*Rubus idaeus*	Provides minerals; balances hormones
2 oz. St. John's wort	*Hypericum perforatum*	Repairs cells; anti-inflammatory herb
2 oz. licorice root	*Glycyrrhiza glabra*	Moistens; soothes digestion; for taste
1 oz. orange peel (organic)	*Citrus aurantium*	For taste; improves digestion
1 oz. hibiscus flower	*Hibiscus sabdariffa*	For taste; nutritive; provides bioflavonoids

Fifteen ounces will last thirty days. Add 1 ounce of the mixture to 4 cups of boiling water in a teapot or container with a well-fitting lid. Let stand for twenty minutes; then strain. Drink 1 to 3 cups daily, hot or cold. *Note:* This mixture uses a small amount of licorice, but if you have high blood pressure, low potassium, or a history of kidney or heart failure, replace it with Siberian ginseng *(Eleutherococcus senticosus)*.

For irregular cycles complicated by heavy bleeding or for spotting between cycles, use one or both of the following formulas instead of those above for erratic timing. These are stronger than the herbal combinations given in Chapter 1 for premenopausal women who are spotting.

CLOSING THE GATES

Extracts	Botanical Names	Actions
4 oz. fresh shepherd's purse herb	*Capsella bursa-pastoris*	Antihemorrhagic; fights infection
2 oz. lady's mantle herb	*Alchemilla vulgaris*	Helps reduce fibroids; protective
2 oz. blue cohosh root	*Caulophyllum thalictroides*	Balances hormones; tones tissue
1 oz. black cohosh root	*Cimicifuga racemosa*	Balances hormones; soothes nerves
1 oz. chasteberry seed	*Vitex agnus-castus*	Harmonizes; balances hormones

Ten ounces will last thirty days. Combine these herbal extracts. Take 1 tablespoon in 1 cup water, juice, or any herb tea every two hours, until bleeding slows down enough; this allows the body time to clot normally and to replace lost blood from reserves. For chronic problems with spotting between cycles, flooding (very heavy flow), and fibroids, take 1 to 2 teaspoons three times a day for a minimum of three months. Consult a health-care provider to help rule out potential dangers associated with menopausal bleeding problems.

Dried Herbs	Botanical Names	Actions
3 oz. chasteberry seed	*Vitex agnus-castus*	Harmonizes; balances hormones
3 oz. sage leaf	*Salvia officinalis*	Lessens excess bleeding; tones tissue
3 oz. partridge berry herb	*Mitchella repens*	Stimulates healing of uterine tissue
3 oz. lady's mantle herb	*Alchemilla vulgaris*	Protects, nourishes uterine tissue
1 1/2 oz. yellow dock root	*Rumex crispus*	Helps elimination; provides iron
1 1/2 oz. cinnamon bark	*Cinnamonum zeylanicum*	Helps digestion; for taste

Fifteen ounces will last thirty days. Add 1 ounce of the mixture to 4 cups of boiling water in a teapot or container with a well-fitting lid. Let stand for fifteen minutes before straining. Drink 1 cup hot or cold three to four times a day.

Nutrition

Wise Food Choices

- In early spring, dandelion leaf in salads or mixed steamed greens
- Pomegranate fruit and seeds
- Dried apricots
- Sesame seeds, tahini (1 tablespoon plain or in prepared dishes, two to three times a week)

Supplements

- Milk thistle (1 tablespoon of seeds daily, ground into powder and sprinkled over cooked grains and salads or blended in soups). May be taken as capsules, two capsules three times a day or three capsules taken two times a day with meals. Standarized silymarin from milk thistle is also available; take as labels suggest.
- Beta-carotene obtained from yellow or orange vegetables is better than from supplements.

Vaginal Thinning and Dryness

During premenopause and menopause, hormonal imbalance may thin or dry the lining of your vagina, causing it to become inflamed or sensitive. If you are experiencing discomfort during intercourse or if vaginal dryness persists despite sexual desire, you may have this condition, called "atrophic vaginitis." To resolve it, you can take herbs to maximize the body's existing estrogen levels from the metabolism of androstenedione produced by the adrenal glands and stored in fat under the skin. Herbal remedies can also optimize progesterone, which helps maintain the necessary balance of sex hormones to keep vaginal tissue healthy. At the same time, you can use herbal remedies to restore the normal, helpful bacterial flora to the mucous membranes lining the vagina. Many of the plants that have this effect contain protective essential oils or other biochemicals that remove inappropriate microbes with few of the side effects of drugs.

Last, but certainly not least, you can work to nourish a sense of emotional well-being within yourself. Vaginal dryness interferes with sex at a time when you may especially need the intimacy of sexual contact to weather challenges to your self-image and identity as a woman. But this condition does not mean your sex life is over: If you want to have sex but you're already feeling friction or irritation, please know that all your hopes do not hang on estrogen alone. Women can have great sex in their seventies if and when they want to. It is yet another false stereotype that libido (sex drive) goes down at menopause. For many, sex becomes a new adventure of body and soul. You may in fact find new appetites or paths to pleasure.

In reality, women find that symptoms associated with hot flashes and vaginal dryness decrease with regular sex. Using sexual energy and releasing it through orgasm, as well as having a healthy attitude toward your changing body, are your best means of controlling the physical discomforts of menopause. Both sex shared with a partner and masturbation stimulate vaginal moisture and brings germ-fighting enzymes into the mucus produced by the glands in the vaginal wall. The blood flow from the head and heart all the way down to the pelvis from happy movements will help restore moisture and dynamic balance in the tissues.

Don't douche unless it helps relieve inflammation and seems absolutely necessary. In most instances you should not need to douche to sanitize or deodorize your vagina. When we are healthy inside our bodies, we are not dirty "down there." Strange odors or itches are a signal that an imbalance is blocking the self-cleaning ways of the body. While vaginal applications may help symptoms such as dryness, thinning of the vaginal walls, or even the infections that may result from vaginal changes, douching may actually create more problems that it solves. One reason is that repeated application of water is in itself eventually drying, making the thinner vaginal wall of menopause (already drier) even more susceptible to infections.

Douching too much rinses away helpful lubrication, such as the enzyme-rich mucus that traps potential microbes. Douching also removes helpful bacterial flora that normally help us maintain an acidic vaginal secretion. This healthy vaginal environment prevents colonization of common opportunistic infections, including yeasts *(Candida)*. Some healing vaginal applications are included in this section, but they are best used for short-term problems or in the context of other changes to clear up an existing condition.

Herbal Medicine

The following formulas prevent or minimize thinning of the vaginal lining by improving circulation, nutrition, and hormonal balance. These recipes utilize the multitalented phytoestrogenic herbs, which, arranged in different "bouquets," have slightly different effects. The following combinations may therefore resemble "Temple Gates Elixir" (see "Sexuality and Vaginal Changes"), but they provide a more broad-based set of actions: They moisturize, strengthen, improve nonspecific immunity, and raise the spirits, especially those of the woman whose Change is well under way.

❦ ————————— MANY SPLENDORED THING ————————— ❦

Extracts	Botanical Names	Actions
4 oz. wild yam root	*Dioscorea villosa*	Anti-inflammatory; supports hormonal balance
2 oz. sarsaparilla root	*Smilax ornata*	Supports lymph, immune, hormonal balance
2 oz. nettle leaf	*Urtica dioica*	Nutritive; aids kidney, liver functions
2 oz. lady's mantle herb	*Alchemilla vulgaris*	Protects and tones vaginal linings; supports hormonal balance
2 oz. lemon balm leaf	*Melissa officinalis*	Antiviral; lifts spirits; for digestion and taste

Twelve ounces will last five weeks. Combine these herbal extracts. Take 1 teaspoon in 1 cup water, juice, or any herb tea in the morning and evening. You can take up to four times a day for quicker results. Best results may be seen after a minimum of two to three months.

Dried Herbs	Botanical Names	Actions
4 oz. lady's mantle herb	*Alchemilla vulgaris*	Tones, tightens vaginal linings
3 oz. red clover flower	*Trifolium pratense*	Phytoestrogens nourish natural estrogen level
3 oz. raspberry leaf	*Rubus idaeus*	Provides calcium; calms nerves; tones tissues
2 oz. rosemary flower, leaf	*Rosmarinus officinalis*	Aromatic oils aid digestion, circulation
2 oz. linden flower	*Tilia* species	Reduces high blood pressure; adds moisture
1 oz. yarrow flower	*Achillea millefolium*	Strengthens circulation; anti-inflammatory

Fifteen ounces will last thirty days. Add 1 ounce of the mixture to 4 cups of boiling water in a teapot or container with a well-fitting lid. Let stand for fifteen minutes and then strain. Drink 1 cup hot or cold, three times a day. Drinking a quart (4 cups) a day brings quicker results; best results are seen in two to three months.

If you've had a chronic vaginal infection, this next herbal combination can be taken safely along with antibiotics if those are considered necessary. Or, this may be used to repair the immune system while preventing a recurrence or clearing up a vaginal infection. It especially helps after repeated courses of antibiotics, which are often prescribed for chronic conditions.

Extracts	Botanical Names	Actions
2 oz. St. John's wort herb	*Hypericum perforatum*	Antiviral; nourishes nerves; antidepressant
2 oz. echinacea root	*Echinacea purpurea*	Stimulates natural immunity, lymphatic function
2 oz. blue cohosh root	*Caulophyllum thalictroides*	Balances hormones; reduces vaginal inflammation
2 oz. black cohosh root	*Cimicifuga racemosa*	Supports natural estrogen level; calms anxiety
1 oz. licorice root	*Glycyrrhiza glabra*	Antiviral; adds moisture; supports hormonal balance
1 oz. fresh shepherd's purse herb	*Capsella bursa-pastoris*	Prevents excess bleeding; reduces infection

Ten ounces will last thirty days. Combine these herbal extracts. Take 1 teaspoon in 1 cup water, juice, or any herb tea every four hours for four days. Then reduce dosage to 1 teaspoon diluted, twice a day in the morning and evening. This compound can be expected to bring some improvement in a few days but more certain results in one to two weeks. It can be taken safely for up to three weeks, by which time reassessment by a care provider is recommended. Some infections are notoriously hard to clear once and for all. If any infection is still present but seems to be responding to the herbs, another three weeks and a retest are wise. In chronic states of infection requiring more than six weeks of herbal therapy, double-check dietary and other recommendations to make sure the cause has been identified and is being handled. If it is, these herbs can be used over the long term by skipping one day each week, up to six months. If desired, replace licorice with sarsaparilla *(Smilax ornata)*.

If you're experiencing vaginal inflammation but there is no infection, use one of the following remedies.

❦ —————————— KISSABLE LIPS POTION —————————— ❦

Extracts	Botanical Names	Actions
4 oz. lady's mantle herb	*Alchemilla vulgaris*	Tones, tightens vaginal linings
4 oz. wild yam root	*Dioscorea villosa*	Anti-inflammatory; supports hormonal, water balance
2 oz. licorice root	*Glycyrrhiza glabra*	Adds moisture; supports hormonal balance
1 oz. yarrow flower	*Achillea millefolium*	Aids as anti-inflammatory; helps circulation
1 oz. nettle leaf	*Urtica dioica*	Nutritive; aids kidney, liver functions

Twelve ounces will last thirty days. Combine these herbal extracts. Take 1 teaspoon in 1 cup water, juice, or any herb tea three times a day after meals. If desired, replace licorice with sage *(Salvia officinalis)*.

❦ —————————— KISSABLE LIPS TEA —————————— ❦

Dried Herbs	Botanical Names	Actions
4 oz. lady's mantle herb	*Alchemilla vulgaris*	Tones, tightens vaginal linings
4 oz. wild yam root	*Dioscorea villosa*	Anti-inflammatory; supports hormonal, water balance
2 oz. licorice root	*Glycyrrhiza glabra*	Adds moisture; supports hormonal balance
1 oz. yarrow flower	*Achillea millefolium*	Aids as anti-inflammatory; helps circulation
1 oz. nettle leaf	*Urtica dioica*	Nutritive; aids kidney, liver functions

Twelve ounces will last just under two weeks. Add 1 ounce of the mixture to 4 cups boiling water in a teapot or container with a well-fitting lid. Let stand for fifteen minutes and then strain. Drink 1 cup hot or cold three times a day. Cover a fourth cup and allow it to cool to room temperature or briefly refrigerate it. Douche once or twice a day with 1/2 to 1 cup while you have inflammation or irritation. If this doesn't clear the problem in two weeks, consider getting a second opinion about the inflammation's cause. If desired, replace licorice with sage *(Salvia officinalis)*.

Sometimes, if bacteria are allowed to thrive in a dry or overdouched vaginal environment, they may cause a bladder infection (cystitis) and ascending kidney infection. Though these conditions require diagnosis by a physician, herbs and other natural treatments can help eliminate them. When the first warning signs of a bladder infection come on (difficulty in urinating or pain on passing urine), prevent their progression by drinking more plain water than usual every day. Cranberry juice can also help: Every two hours for two to four days, as needed, drink an 8-ounce glass of juice to which has been added a pinch of baking soda (not baking powder). While using this remedy, you must limit yourself to a sugar-free liquid diet.

If water or cranberry juice isn't helping, try the following herbal tea. Herbal teas work better for bladder infections than concentrated extracts or capsules because the water helps flush out invading organisms from the kidneys and bladder without too much extra effort. You will need to frequently visit the bathroom during this cleansing process.

❧ ——— Slow Flow Go Tea ——— ❧

Dried Herbs	Botanical Names	Actions
4 oz. bearberry leaf	*Arctostaphylos uva-ursi*	Helps disinfect urinary tract
3 oz. echinacea root	*Echinacea purpurea*	Fights microorganisms directly; increase natural resistance
3 oz. cramp bark	*Viburnum opulus*	Reduces painful urination, spasms
2 oz. linden flower	*Tilia* species	Relaxes nerves; for circulation
2 oz. parsley leaf	*Petroselinum crispus*	Helps kidneys flush out urine

Fourteen ounces will last three weeks. Add 1/2 ounce of the mixture to 3 cups boiling water in a teapot or container with a well-fitting lid. Let stand for fifteen minutes and then strain. Drink 1 cup hot or cold every two hours for the first three days; then reduce tea to 1 cup three times a day. It may not take all twenty-one days to feel better, but finish up the tea whether or not you have symptoms—your bladder and immune system will thank you. After these three weeks, your kidneys will have been supported so well that your skin may feel smoother, a bonus for not stopping the tea too soon. If you substitute fresh organic parsley for dried, use 1 standard organic grocery-store bunch (about a large handful) every three days (one-third bunch per day). *Note:* If a repeated or severe infection accompanied by fever or other signs does not respond well to herbs in two to three days, contact a qualified health-care provider or experienced herbalist.

Nutrition

Wise Food Choices

- Use garlic, a source of zinc and other relevant nutrients.
- The wide variety of whole foods that are rich in phytosterols help alleviate vaginal atrophy. These include beans and legumes, sprouted seeds, nuts, pomegranates, dates, carrots, yams, real licorice candy, and real ale (with hops).
- Nutrients from whole foods accelerate the elimination of symptoms as well as prevent recurrences. Please see "Herbs and Nutrition in Menopause," earlier in this chapter.
- Avoid sugar and refined and processed foods. Even honey, maple syrup, and an excess of sweet fruit juices may interfere with the body's ability to fight the infection, especially when vaginitis is associated with chronic yeast.
- Eat sour fruits (lemon, grapefruit, cranberries, plums) in season. Drink one glass of cranberry juice (naturally sweetened with white grape juice and diluted with an equal part of pure water; avoid brands containing glucose and corn syrup) per day.

Supplements

- Vitamin E can help with vaginal problems, especially thinning and dryness. In a study of forty-seven women who were taking 500 I.U. of vitamin E per day, two-thirds were helped; half of this group who had vaginal lesions due to thinning or drying were healed.
- Zinc helps heal inflammation and tears in the vaginal wall, and it's useful for other wounds, too.

In Addition

- You can participate in intercourse as long as you do not have an infection and it feels enjoyable. Sex stimulates secretion of mucus from the vaginal walls.
- Practice Kegel exercises five minutes a day. See "Kegels" box in Chapter 1, "Premenopause."
- Natural lubricants can make a big difference. These are not simply herbal versions of petroleum jelly. Licorice, calendula, St. John's wort, and comfrey heal minor tears, soften and moisten, fight infection, and lessen inflammation. Wild yam oil is the basis for many natural creams used specifically in menopause for improving vaginal lubrication. The herb's plant sterols (phytosterols) have a beneficial effect on the vagina and a woman's entire system, but there is no certainty that wild yam or other herbal preparations with phytosterols for vaginal or skin massage increase estrogen. They do have remarkable anti-inflammatory and healing properties regardless of the exact biochemical mechanism. Many natural lubricants are available for sale in herb shops and natural-food stores and from mail-order businesses; see "Resources."
- You may want to make an all-natural herbal salve; see "More Love Vaginal Salve" box in Chapter 1. Making your own salve is a great way to incorporate herbs into your daily life. At first it may be messy, but it is always fun and smells terrific.
- A still easier way to combine healing herbs for your vagina is to add essential oils from plants (not blends or perfumes of flowers) to liquid vitamin E oil. See "Sexuality and Vaginal Changes" in Chapter 1, "Premenopause."
- The following is a soothing vaginal application for inflammation that does not dry tissues. Mix 2 tablespoons aloe vera gel with 1/4 cup sterilized water (boiled and cooled to a comfortably cool temperature—not just from the tap). Whisk or stir briskly until the gel is mixed well into the water. There will be some clumps. Use 1 to 2 tablespoons at a time; cover and refrigerate the rest. Spread the labia with the clean fingers of one hand, and apply the mixture with clean fingers of the other hand. Insert a few fingerfuls into the canal without forcing. Gently massage it into the vaginal opening and outer labia, wherever extra soothing is needed. Wash hands well; wear old underwear or relax where you can wear none at all for an hour or two. Repeat twice daily up to a week; then repeat every once in a while as needed. This mixture works well when used over a few months, alternating as desired with "More Love Vaginal Salve," described in Chapter 1.
- Try a stronger herbal douche (see box). This formula is *for external use only*. Combining vulnerary (wound-healing) teas and an antimicrobial essential oil, it helps with vaginal infections caused by menopausal changes rather than simply rehydrating dry or thin vaginal membranes. It may seem silly to

Herbal Douche for Vaginal Infections

Ingredients

5 oz. yarrow flower *(Achillea millefolium)*
5 oz. calendula flower *(Calendula officinalis)*
4 drops essential oil of marjoram per cup of tea (see below)

This mixture helps the vaginal tissues regain immune resistance and moisture balance; as a bonus, its aromatherapy value is soothing to the nerves. Ten ounces will last ten days. Add 1 ounce of the herb mixture to 2 cups of boiling water, cover, and steep for forty-five minutes or until cool to the touch. Do not add the essential oil when the tea is still hot or it will evaporate and be less effective. After the tea is cool to the touch, strain; then add 4 drops of essential oil to 6 to 8 ounces of strong herb tea. The marjoram oil works best when dispersed thoroughly in the herb tea, so stir or shake well. Pour into a sterilized douche bag, available from drugstores and supermarkets in the pharmacy section.

Sitting on a toilet, lean back and insert the applicator about an inch or two into the vaginal canal (there's no need to go deeper). Holding the bag up and squeezing *gently,* let the herbal liquid flow in. It isn't necessary to hold the herbal liquid in: Let it rinse out of the vagina and flow into the toilet bowl. You don't have to rinse afterward because the herbs have an anti-inflammatory, antimicrobial, and astringent action on the vaginal walls—not drying, but toning and moistening. Sterilize the douche bag and applicator with a mild antiseptic and boiling water after every use. Dry the equipment before storing it. Repeat application once or twice daily, depending on the infection's severity and the duration of relief. Continue for no more than ten days. Whether or not antibiotics or other medication are needed, you can safely use this douche in combination with "The Chalice Well," described previously.

say "external use only" when we all know the vagina is located inside, but it means that the mixture is not to be taken by mouth because it includes a strong essential oil.

- Yogurt is an old standby of kitchen medicine that sometimes works but is mainly for minor yeast infections. Use plain, live culture, organic yogurt (not the flavored kind with fruit at the bottom). Apply a teasoon at a time, liberally swabbing it on reddened, sore spots with clean fingers. Wear a panty liner, flannel menstrual pad, or old underwear. The yogurt stays in most easily while you sleep or lie horizontally.

- Goldenseal is a popular herbal remedy that is powerful enough to be misused. Now often overused, this antimicrobial herb was at one time the best remedy Western herbalists had for restoring mucous membranes. It is most effective when taken orally in small amounts (10 to 30 drops in 1/4 cup water three times a day for fourteen days) and used as a vaginal douche (1 ounce of powdered herb to 1 pint water; see the standard preparation

Meditation for Emotional Balance

Have someone read this to you, or play a tape recording of yourself reading it. If you record this, you may wish to leave a silent pause of twenty-five seconds or more where asterisks (*) appear. The entire meditation can last as briefly as three minutes or as long as an hour—it's up to you and the time you have available. Close your eyes for the meditation.

Breathe deeply. Relax any tension you may feel in your jaw or neck. *

Put aside any thoughts you may have for just this moment; allow your inner eye to gaze on a landscape of symbol—geometric shapes, meanings expressed in color or pictures that are not logical yet are true for you. Because this journey is in your imagination, you can stop at any time, undisturbed, still in charge of your Self. Breathe in deeply and breathe out slowly.

In your mind's eye, take all your attention to the center of your body—the very center. It is about halfway down your body, about 4 inches below your navel. There, almost invisible because it is not truly physical, a seed of pure energy vibrates. This seed crystal of your essence vibrates with every color of the light spectrum, flashing red, then the orange of a harvest moon, solar yellow, garden green, sky blue, midnight blue, and indescribable violet. *

In your imagination, let your inner eye see the vibration of red, so deeply red that it could be the seed from which all red grows. It is the red of the rose that can take your breath away. The rose perfumes our world with a wild and cultured love whose language is fragrance.

Breathe and relax. Let this rose red open before your inner eye into a bud of palest pink. Watch and continue to breathe evenly as it deepens to a warm pink blush, followed by the deepest burgundy of a mature bloom. *

Rich red, the vibration of blood, river of life. Now rose colors from your center diffuse through your every cell, cascading like a waterfall of burgundy rose petals, nourishing your womb, your ovaries—even if they have been removed. This wise vibration nourishes the body memory of your perfectly integrated creative center. Let it fall and rise to flow to every layer of tissue, kissing every living cell. This red flows to heal any wounds you may have received; let them receive healing, forgiveness, your compassionate and full attention. *

With your inner eyes you may see this red glow brighten and dim, ebb and flow, as it brings wisdom. Its vibration responds to the pull of the moon, yet this rose red will not flow out of you to nourish the Earth or even to mother a new little life. It is kept inside for nourishing your being, birthing your renewed woman's spirit. When it no longer flows in rosy rivers outside of us, it flows mysteriously within our blood to nourish deep wellsprings within our Earth, our bodies, the peak of our beings. You are connected to the red center of our planetary body. Fiery energy from the timeless internal ocean of Earth's central flame rises through layers of earth to bring you living rose red, blood red, fiery red life for the work you have taken on. *

Gently bring your attention back to your whole body, and breathe evenly. When you feel ready, open your eyes.

described in "Herbal Preparations." Because goldenseal is now endangered in the wild from overharvesting, its use is best reserved for damaged mucous membranes infected with stubborn, resistant microbes that cannot be eliminated by conventional methods. If you have a real need, it may help to take 1 capsule (250 milligrams) of goldenseal powder with an 8-ounce glass of lady's mantle and yarrow tea (equal parts, standard preparation), for up to three months. Goldenseal is not at its best when taken every day for this long, so after you take it daily for three weeks, reduce dosage to two days on, one day off.

Note: Goldenseal must be avoided in pregnancy because it can cause uterine contractions. Change of Life babies do get born, so keep in mind that menopause includes the possibility of a pregnancy. For adults who have been kicking around for a while, this immune-stimulating herb safely and effectively eliminates germs and fights against immune dysfunction. For babies and tiny children, it is too strong.

- Meditation and visualization can bring profound healing to the physical body by uniting it with the nonphysical aspects of ourselves. See the accompanying box for one suggested visualization.

Changing Appearance of Skin and Hair

You'll notice that your hair and skin become drier at menopause. This change is not solely due to declining estrogen but also to shifting levels of nutrients and hormones in general. Now, more than ever, you need to eat well, optimize circulation to the skin and scalp, and protect the outer surface of your body in order to avoid dry skin and hair.

The herbs for strengthening bone resiliency and suggestions for preventing osteoporosis also help with hair and skin. Dry hair and skin also can be conditioned by regular use of moisturizing plants and oils. Aromatic plants with oils—for example, rosemary, sage, lemon balm, and lemon grass—make good daily hair rinses. Dry or mature skin responds well to the moisturizing herbs, especially comfrey, chamomile, sandalwood, and calendula. These are also called "vulnerary," or wound healing, because they speed the body's self-repair of scratches, burns, rashes, wounds, and other "vulnerable" places on the surface of the scalp and skin.

Women have been using herbs for hair care for millennia, including less-usual cosmetic aids such as black walnut, cloves, coffee, and henna, and extracted oils such as olive, jojoba, and vitamin E. The beauty of getting on in years is that skin actually softens unless we callous it with rough treatment or overexposure to chemicals and sun. An old lady's face is wonderfully soft, like a baby's. No matter what we have done with our skin and hair in the past decades, a six-month regimen of the following extract and/or tea nourishes body and soul, from the inside out.

Herbal Medicine

Extracts	Botanical Names	Actions
4 oz. wild yam root	*Dioscorea villosa*	Nourishes skin; anti-inflammatory; hormonal tonic
4 oz. rosemary flower, leaf	*Rosmarinus officinalis*	Optimizes circulation, assimilation of nutrients
1 oz. nettle leaf	*Urtica dioica*	Mineralizing nutritive; tonic for good elimination
1 oz. licorice root	*Glycyrrhiza glabra*	Moistening; helps liver balance hormones; for taste

Ten ounces will last thirty days. Combine these herbal extracts. Take 1 teaspoon in 1 cup water, diluted juice, or herb tea in the morning and evening. If desired, licorice may be replaced with sarsaparilla *(Smilax ornata)*.

GRANDMOTHER'S KISS TEA

Dried Herbs	Botanical Names	Actions
5 oz. wild yam root	*Dioscorea villosa*	Nourishes skin; anti-inflammatory; hormonal tonic
4 oz. rosemary flower, leaf	*Rosmarinus officinalis*	Optimizes circulation, assimilation of nutrients
2 oz. nettle leaf	*Urtica dioica*	Mineralizing nutritive; tonic for good elimination
2 oz. licorice root	*Glycyrrhiza glabra*	Moistening; helps liver balance hormones; for taste
2 oz. lemon grass leaf	*Cymbopogon* species	Moistening; for taste

Fifteen ounces will last thirty days. Add 1/2 ounce of the mixture to 3 1/2 cups of boiling water in a teapot or container with a well-fitting lid. Let stand for fifteen minutes and then strain. Drink 1 cup hot or cold three times a day. If you prefer, sip tea throughout the day or drink two large glasses twice a day, but be sure you drink 3 cups a day. If desired, licorice may be replaced with sarsaparilla *(Smilax ornata)*.

My favorite external herbal formula for dry hair is a combination I learned from two beautiful Moroccan herbal students. It can be used to condition or naturally tint the hair and is easy to create variations with each batch. The main variation for many readers may be the use or avoidance of henna powder *(Lawsonia inermis)*. Henna comes in red, neutral, and other colors, and though this Egyptian cosmetic herb is useful, it takes one or two times of experimenting with the henna-powder-and-water mud pack to feel that you know what you are doing, and the results vary, naturally. A little goes a long way. Overuse of henna (every few months for two or more years) is drying to hair, especially if it is just mixed with water. The other herbs and oils in this combination minimize that problem, but when in doubt, leave the henna out. Enjoy!

❦———————SAMIA AND FATIMA'S DIAMANDA SPECIAL———————❦

Dried Herbs	Botanical Names	Actions
2 oz. rosemary leaf, flower	*Rosmarinus officinalis*	Conditions; darkens gray
1 oz. horsetail leaves	*Equisetum arvense*	Coats hair shaft with minerals
1 oz. chamomile flower	*Matricaria recutita*	Volatile oils nourish, add moisture
1 oz. nettle leaf	*Urtica dioica*	Conditions hair and scalp
1/2 oz. black walnut hulls	*Juglans nigra*	Darkens, covers gray
1/2 oz. clove powder	*Eugenia caryophyllata*	Volatile oils nourish, add moisture
1/2 oz. ground coffee	*Coffea* species	Volatile oils nourish, add moisture
Hot water (not quite boiling) sufficient to make a paste		
1 tbsp. (or up to 4 oz.) of olive oil		Keeps henna from over-drying hair
Optional: 1 to 4 oz. henna powder	*Lawsonia inermis*	Conditions hair; colors cover gray with neutral, red, brown pigments, or other desired color

Other items you may need: mirror, drinking water, clock, comb, glass or ceramic bowl, plastic gloves, shower cap, at least one old towel, wash cloth, mild shampoo, moisturizer or facial cream.

Grind the herbs to a fine powder in a blender or one at a time in a coffee grinder. Remove as many stems as you have the patience to sift out. Stir powders together.

In a nonmetal covered container (glass or ceramic bowl with a lid or a salad bowl and a plate), pour the hot water on the herbs and soak, covered, for ten minutes.

Position mirror, drinking water, clock, comb, bowl, plastic gloves, and at least one old towel near the sink. Cover the surrounding floor (an old shower curtain makes a good floor covering). Lightly shampoo hair; towel dry. Place a thin line of moisturizer or facial cream around the hairline, including the tops of your ears, to avoid staining facial skin. Stir olive oil into wet herb mixture to get a smooth paste of oatmeal consistency. The mixture shouldn't run through the fingers or crumble into dry lumps. Add spoonfuls of water or oil to get the right consistency. If it gets too wet, add more powdered dry herbs.

Divide clean, damp hair into sections and apply this herb goo, massaging it into the scalp. It may make a mess, so go slowly and have fun. When hair is covered with an even thickness, roots to ends, swish a few spoonfuls of warm water in the henna bowl to make a little herb-flecked "tea" to pat on or pour over the mud pack on your head. This ensures that the mixture soaks down evenly to the roots of your hair.

Use a damp wash cloth frequently to wipe any drips from your neck and face. Cover your hair with an old towel or shower cap. The herb mixture shouldn't get dry over the next fifteen to ninety minutes, so keep the scalp wet—if necessary, by covering the hair first with a shower cap or plastic bag or by periodically changing to a new hot, wet towel. Keep drinking water or herb teas as you may not notice that you are becoming dehydrated from the warmth. After fifteen minutes, rinse out a test strand. Don't worry—this isn't like using plain henna. Once I fell asleep like this for four hours and my hair didn't go orange, but it sure was deeply conditioned! Depending on your test strand, gauge your remaining time—the longer the time, the deeper the color and/or conditioning. After one to two hours, or when you have had enough, or the weight of the mud pack and towel tires your neck muscles, remove the towel and/or shower cap and get in the shower. Rinse out the herbs with plain water before using *dilute* mild shampoo. Then massage shampoo into the hair and scalp with gentle motions. When fully lathered, rinse and repeat as needed. You will probably wash your hair several times; if you like, condition as usual. The first day your hair may feel dry, but from the second day on it will shine.

Repeat once every six to twelve weeks as desired but not more than four to six times a year, total. Henna is a stain, after all, and overuse can cause eventual allergic sensitivity—the irritation is your body's way of letting you know it's no longer okay to use so much. This same herb conditioning can be repeated without henna for one or two hours as often as you like.

Aromatic Skin and Hair Rinse

Ingredients

1 oz. comfrey leaf or root
1/2 oz. chamomile flower
1/4 oz. calendula flower
15 drops essential oil of sandalwood
5 drops essential oil of rosemary
3 drops essential oil of lemon grass

Steep the herbs in 2 pints (16 cups) boiling water, covered, for forty minutes; strain when warm but not hot into a clean plastic (not glass) bottle. Add all essential oils, shake well to mix, and shake again before each use. Keep in bath or shower, as a final rinse or alternative to shampoo during dry spells in winter or summer. Can be splashed as desired on face or body, massaged in instead of lotion. Since the preservative power of the essential oils fades as the oils slowly evaporate through the bottle, use each batch in two to four weeks, discarding any sour-smelling portion. In warm climates, refrigerate the mixture and take out only a week's worth at a time. A final note: Trust your nose. You may like this for years or change your opinion of it after a few months. If you want to change the formula, use different herbs or substitute other aromatherapy-quality oils. By all means, please yourself! You are the best and only real judge of what your body chemistry responds to in a healing way.

Nutrition

Wise Food Choices

- Eat soy foods unless you are allergic to them.
- Drink 1 teaspoon of flax seed meal stirred into a glass of water once a day for at least two months.
- Eat a quarter or half avocado twice a week in salads or garlic vegetable dip (guacamole is great but not with bags of tortilla chips).
- Eat one or two pieces of organic fruit per day (choose fruits in season), followed with water or herb tea.
- For better blood sugar, appetite control, energy levels, and metabolism, eat fruit with 1 teaspoon raw sunflower seeds or five to ten raw, unsalted almonds. Chew slowly.
- Avoid all heated, hydrogenated, or partially hydrogenated oils and fats (margarine, bakery items).
- Avoid refined sugars.

Supplements

- Omega-3 capsules, as directed on label
- Evening primrose oil, 3 capsules three times a day for one to six months

In Addition

- Women in their thirties and forties may feel ultrasensitive about how they are perceived. Your looks do not "go," but they do change. Turn your back on powerful media messages aimed at your vanity and your purse. A truly feminine spirit at this time of life is more similar to a mature tigress—who can be serenely contented or powerfully pissed off—than to a sappy TV mannequin.
- Define beauty for yourself. White, silver, or gray hair is beautiful. Set it with silver hair combs and get it conditioned, braided, or cut in a new way you've always wanted to see on yourself.
- Make an aromatic rinse for your skin and hair (see box on previous page).
- Exercise, exercise, exercise! It sweats out impurities, decreases tension, optimizes circulation, and releases hormones for immune health and an uplifted mood.
- Take saunas as often as you wish or can tolerate.

Chapter 3

HORMONE
REPLACEMENT THERAPY

The idea of hormone replacement therapy (HRT) and estrogen replacement therapy (ERT)—that all symptoms of menopause can be reversed or avoided with hormone supplements—makes sense only if you believe that menopause is a deficiency of estrogen. Despite their general acceptance by the American medical profession, however, they are not always the right choice, nor are they necessary for every woman. HRT and ERT are not really therapies at all, but drug treatments—powerful, concentrated hormones taken during and after menopause. This chapter discusses the pros and cons of HRT, ERT, and "natural" sources of hormones. It also provides herbal remedies that you can safely take along with HRT and that help you slowly come off it.

HRT is a combination of estrogen and progesterone. Some progesterone is needed to help continue the monthly shedding of the uterine lining, and it prevents some of the risks of cancer associated with use of estrogen alone, although it does not eliminate all of them. ERT, which does not include progesterone, is not as commonly prescribed because it is linked to cancer of the uterine lining, and so is primarily given to women who have undergone removal of the uterus. Studies in which only estrogen was given show that it may help the heart and bones, but these findings are not absolute and final. There is less proof that estrogen and progesterone, the more usually prescribed combination, work as well at protecting us from heart attacks and osteoporosis. One problem with lab studies is that they cannot reflect the different ways a set dose of estrogen acts in different women. Variables include diet (vegetarian, low-fat, meat-eating, fiber content, and so forth), body weight, alcohol sensitivity, and liver function, as well as types of intestinal bacteria, time between eating and eliminating (transit time), enzyme activity, and age. The several kinds of estrogen that are made naturally in the body or that are converted in metabolism make a big difference, too. Studies are not the gospel truth, whether we like what they say or disagree with the results. All are worth consideration; few are worth banking on.

Advantages of HRT

According to reviews of medical literature by the National Women's Health Network, HRT may be a wise choice in menopause for (1) relieving the symptoms of extreme hot flashes; (2) helping insomnia caused by night sweats; (3) lessening severe risk of osteoporosis; and (4) preventing extreme vaginal dryness. The U.S. Food and Drug Administration (FDA) has approved it only for preventing osteoporosis. In my opinion, HRT is useful only when natural methods have not been able to alleviate the problems a woman is having; she understands that HRT will suppress her symptoms, not "cure" her; she knows the risks of taking hormones and can accept those risks; and the prescription improves her quality of life. Drugs are not "bad" compared to all-natural herbs: A woman's well-being is more important than moral judgments about whether it came from natural approaches or synthetic hormones. A well-informed woman may choose to avoid or take HRT, and even to come gradually off hormones safely, should that be her desire.

Disadvantages of HRT

The disadvantages of HRT are many. You should not use it if you have high blood pressure, uterine fibroids, diabetes, estrogen-dependent breast cancer now or in the past, any significant liver or gallbladder disease, or cardiovascular disease; nor should you use it during pregnancy. Replacing hormones the body is trying to decrease goes against the natural process, especially if you are reasonably healthy, so if you value the natural experience of menopause rather than want to "stop the clock" by artificial means, HRT may not be for you. Then there's the bother of running out to fill the prescription and remembering to take it. HRT also means higher costs and more required medical visits. Though it is rarely done, in some cases doctors recommend an annual D & C (dilation and curettage), a procedure to scrape the uterus. HRT can cause incomplete shedding of the uterine lining, so if a woman has persistent bleeding, an endometrial sample may lead a doctor to recommend an annual D & C to lower the risks of disease and cancer of the uterine lining. Sometimes a D & C is necessary even for women taking combined estrogen and progesterone.

To continue their bleeding cycles, women are usually prescribed Premarin (estrogen) (0.625 milligram every day for days 1 to 25 of the cycle), followed by Provera (progestin) (2.5, 5, or even 10 milligrams for days 13 to 25). Though the higher dosages are now reserved mainly for women under age fifty-five, there are cases of women reaching seventy-five who still have a period every month. Commonly, but not always, women over age fifty-five are switched to a continuous cycle of Premarin (0.625 milligram every day) and Provera (2.5 milligrams every day), so periods do not continue, although estrogen-dependent fibroids, benign or other breast lumps, and menstrual migraines stay actively stimulated by the hormones. These conditions, as well as mood swings, may even worsen. The Centers for Disease Control found in 1991 that for a woman on HRT, the risk of cancer of the uterus or breast is calculated to go up to 30 percent after ten years, and this risk continues to rise the longer a woman stays on HRT.

Women are not routinely told about the effects on all parts of the body from taking hormones made outside their body, whether they are using it in the form of pill, injection, cream, suppository, or patch. Some women are better, some feel the same, some are worse with the drug, suffering especially from depression and uncontrolled hot flashes. The rest of the body experiences these effects even if the uterus, ovaries, or both are removed before HRT begins.

Something else we are often not told: The most popular estrogen used in HRT comes from pregnant mare's urine (Premarin); other types may be totally synthetic. The ugly truth about how the urine is "farmed" raises ethical questions for every woman who considers herself caring and compassionate. Synthetic hormones have previously proven to be a two-edged sword for women's health. For example, DES, a popular drug used to ease morning sickness in pregnant women, now linked to breast and uterine cancer and birth defects in developing female offspring, was not associated with these problems until more than twenty years after its use began, despite large numbers of prescriptions to women.

HRT may ease signs and symptoms, but high costs in health are likely over time because many women stay on HRT for years. HRT has not been proven safe and effective for all women. There are no studies on large enough groups of women over time to get reliable, unbiased data (unless we count the current generations of women on HRT as an experiment in progress). Research regarding risks to women sometimes exclude women who used the birth control pill or DES, so the safety of their use of HRT remains questionable. The next generation of potential HRT patients will also have been exposed to the Pill at a younger age and may well experience different effects on their reproductive health as years go by. Every few years, warnings about the medically accepted practice and dosage tables change, usually with amounts being lowered.

Estrogen does apparently lower the risk of osteoporosis and heart attacks, but, just like the Pill, it also increases the risk of high blood pressure, emboli-causing strokes, and cancer. Furthermore, estrogen may cause unpredictable complications in older women, who, having weathered more medical incidents than younger women, may therefore be more susceptible to estrogen's negative health effects. For a woman who took the Pill in the 1960s or 1970s and is now on HRT, the heavy risk combination ought to be a concern. This is not meant to scare you but rather to encourage you to ask questions, be skeptical of easy answers, and to request your physician to show you evidence (research, summaries) about HRT's proven benefits that relate to you personally.

A Swedish study (1988) reported that the estrogen-progesterone combination was more effective than estrogen alone against hot flashes and sweating but increased a negative mood or mental outlook. This, they concluded, made it unusable. Women reported a drop in sex enjoyment on HRT, an increase in tension, and worsened depression. Now let's just stop and think about that. For which common symptoms is HRT prescribed?

In an Australian review of several studies on the psychological effects of synthetic progesterone (progestin) added to estrogen in menopausal medication, the reviewers note that 85 percent of the women in one study asked to be taken off the study and the medication because of side effects that included withdrawal bleeding that was worse than their former periods and out-of-control mood swings. Progesterones added to estrogens gave PMS-like symptoms, including simultaneous depression and agitation. These side effects are pretty common, so now if women on HRT report them, the progesterone is what is dropped first. Some doctors instead advocate the use of natural progesterone instead of estrogen for improving bone density, reducing hot flashes, and optimizing other aspects of health during and after menopause.

Often, women are not told about the link between progestin and heart disease. Normally, women are prescribed estrogen to lower the risk of heart disease, but it must be followed with progestin for at least seven to ten days per cycle—some doctors say fourteen days. Otherwise, the unopposed estrogen can cause problems. As long ago as 1989, however, a Consensus Conference determined that the use of progestin resulted in an increased risk of heart disease.

The benefits of HRT on cardiovascular risks are unclear in natural menopause, but these claimed benefits are even less clear for women who are experiencing premature menopause, especially when it is due to surgery. These women may require HRT on the basis of a quality-of-life principle, but because they must take it longer than usual, dosages ought to be in the lowest amounts possible. Even for women with surgical or medically caused menopause, natural remedies may provide ample support but fewer long-term risks.

Some Background

When and how did ERT and HRT become the standard drug approach to menopause? In the late 1960s, supported by chauvinistic preconceptions, estrogen was a "wonder drug" that exploited women's fears about aging, which included losing our socially accepted role as a potentially reproductive girlfriend, wife, and mother or the "alternative" role of the ever-sexy femme fatale. To judge from popular media, the dominant cultural bias still accepts the stereotype of menopausal women as neurotic, whiny, asexual, and unattractive. If a woman has laugh lines around her eyes or is no longer willing to put up or shut up, she is ready, according to "modern" Western culture, to be put out to pasture. Older women are being medicated for being their own age. Advertisements for HRT in medical journals frequently depict women who do not use HRT as decrepit and gray; women who use it are air-brushed, pink-lipped, and kissed by men. Meanwhile, silver-haired men with paunches are dashing around with women the age of their daughters—and that midlife crisis is still applauded even as our dominant culture jokes about it. The decline of testosterone and other male sex hormones taking place between forty and sixty has not been pinpointed for treatment like a woman's end of monthly cycles, but both transitions are real. While many women and men today are admirably redefining social roles, the thrust of our Western culture gives only lip service to older women's rights, and that's not good enough.

By the time estrogen became one of the top five drugs prescribed in the United States in the mid-1970s, rates for cancer of the uterine lining, ovaries, and breasts had increased five to fourteen times higher than normal and incidences of uterine fibroids, fibrocystic breast lumps, and gallbladder disease were far higher. These last conditions especially affect Native American women and women with high cholesterol, as well as women who are twenty pounds overweight or more because body fat creates more estrogen.

When a link between the use of estrogen and cancers of the ovaries, uterus, and breasts was cautiously "suggested," prescriptions plummeted. Pharmaceutical companies had increased production, but their warehouses stayed full. Public relations firms and women doctors hired by the companies flooded television and women's magazines with carefully worded ads and new items claiming that the risks were exaggerated. Then women's health groups and physicians worked with the FDA to demand warning labels on estrogen prescriptions. In 1979 the National Institutes of Health rejected drug manufacturers' claims current in marketing at that time, especially as they related to HRT's psychological and physical benefits. The NIH accepted the use of HRT only for hot flashes and vaginal dryness. In the end, drug companies shifted to using combined HRT rather than ERT for women with reproductive organs, to decrease the risk of uterine cancer. However, the combination of estrogen and progesterone can result in unpleasant withdrawal bleeding and incomplete uterine shedding.

Hormones from Herbs

There are some common misconceptions about herbal sources of hormones among natural health-care providers, women using herbal remedies, and conventional medical personnel. The fact is, human or animal hormones, including estrogen, progesterone, and DHEA (dihydroepiandrosterone), are not found in herbs, except in tiny amounts or in different vegetable versions. (DHEA is a steroidal hormone from the adrenal glands, like cortisol, that has broad-ranging effects on health, probably including prevention of osteoporosis.) Some manufacturers claim that wild yam, for instance, is converted into the hormones a menopausal woman needs, but there is no evidence that it can be synthesized into natural hormones in the body. Wild yam is a time-honored anti-inflammatory and adrenal remedy for menopausal women, but not as a raw source of human hormone replacements. What herbs *do* contain are plant hormones (phytoestrogens, phytosterols, and others) with hormonal-type effects. They only behave like hormones as they lock into human cell receptors. We know something, but not everything, about these effects in women, because for thousands of years women have been using the plants or whole-plant extracts with fairly predictable effects. The synthesized hormones made from raw material in herbs, such as the DHEA made from diosgenin (extracted from wild yam), do not occur like those in nature. "Natural progesterone" made from wild yam or other herb extracts is a pharmaceutically manipulated hormone used for its druglike effects. Products that include it may help women with symptoms, but it is misleading to call them "natural." They are not.

The difference between vegetable, animal, and synthetic hormones is as simple as the difference between eggs and egg substitutes. If you are not interested in biochemistry, feel free to skip this section.

Biochemically speaking, human sex steroids (sex hormones) are of three kinds: *pregnanes,* which provide the basic compound for making all kinds of progestins and corticoids; *androstanes*, for making androgens (hormones associated with masculine secondary sex characteristics in both sexes); and *estranes,* which the body can make into all types of estrogen. All three types of sex steroids have the same basic "building block" with different numbers of carbon molecules, in slightly different arrangements. Minor chemical differences translate into huge sexual differences in humans. Two carbons more or less is the difference between a man and a woman.

We can find some compounds in plants that are related to human sex steroids. All plants contain vegetable versions of some estrogenlike hormones for the plant's growth and reproduction. These are not identical to human hormones, but there is some related activity. Sterol glycosides are one example of plant hormones. The group found in ginseng *(Panax ginseng)* are called "ginsenosides." The ginsenosides can have a stimulating effect on our hormones. Sometimes this stimulation is good in menopause; sometimes it worsens health conditions. This is why herbalists always repeat ad nauseam that we have to see each woman rather than prescribe an herb for a condition. In a limited book of this kind, there are several herb formulas for women to choose from if there is no herbalist nearby.

Triterpenoid saponins are a second example of herbal hormones that have an influence on our hormone balance and health—for example, the compound glycyrrhizin found in licorice root *(Glycyrrhiza glabra)*. The whole plant taken medicinally is weakly estrogenic in its effects and has other hormonal effects described in the "Materia Medica" section and in formulas including licorice root. A third type of herbal hormonal compound that has become familiar to many menopausal women today is the steroidal saponin, such as diosgenin from wild yam *(Dioscorea villosa)*. It is anti-inflammatory and may have a beneficial influence on the production of hormones though it contains no human hormones. Traditional herbal practice can predict low toxicity with all these whole plants since less important chemicals buffer or moderate the hormonal stimulation, reducing the likelihood of side effects. An isolated chemical from the plants is predictably less safe.

Essential oils are another type of plant compound biochemically related to sex hormones. These are often isolated (from the plant's fiber or chlorophyll, for instance) but are used in very small amounts. Their strong effects on balancing hormones have been known for much longer than pharmaceutical or synthetic hormone derivatives. This is partly because essential oils share a fundamental property bridging plant and animal life processes: cholesterol. Naturally occurring cholesterol is a basic building block for hormones in mammals. Cholesterol also forms essential oils in certain plants, though it isn't cholesterol by the time it is part of a plant. As modern food labeling keeps reminding us, plant oils are by definition "cholesterol free." The aromas of these herbs or their essential oils affect mammals powerfully. In therapeutic herbal medicine, traditional use of essential oils in context usually stimulates better internal regulation of sex hormones. This is not the same as simply stimulating an increase of sex hormones. An example of hormone-balancing essential oil is clary sage *(Salvia sclarea)*.

It makes sense that vegetables do not normally contain the same sex hormones for flowering and dropping seed that animals need for their reproduction. On the other hand, a few known plants can yield a variation that is amazingly close. The date palm *(Phoenix dactylifera)*, associated since ancient times with fertility in camels, women, and other mammals, contains a small quantity of estrone, especially during that desert tree's natural reproductive season. But other than examples such as that, phytoestrogens (estrogenlike compounds found in certain plants) fall into the two main groups identified so far. I've already talked about three categories in the first main group: the steroidal glycosides, triterpenoid saponins, and steroidal saponins found in herbs such as ginseng, licorice, and wild yam. These compounds related to sterol and cholesterol are one main group of phytoestrogens. The second main group contains the isoflavone type of phytoestrogens. Formononetin, a common isoflavone, is found in red clover *(Trifolium pratense)* and many other herbs. The bitter herb hops *(Humulus lupulus)* contains far higher amounts of formononetin than red clover and other pea family plants, and it contains high amounts of estronelike phytoestrogens. But, lucky for us, we do not usually eat hops as a main course or even as a side dish of vegetables. Nature set it up so that certain powerful herbs (like hops) are too nasty tasting to eat on a regular basis, thus preventing the likelihood of problems from arising.

Many women are told to stop taking estrogenic herbs because their doctors do not understand what experienced herbalists know about these herbs. Doctors are trained to think of estrogenlike compounds as having only one effect. Estrogenic herbs have been shown to have paradoxical effects. Traditional women's herbal remedies that have helped female problems caused by high estrogen are known to contain phytoestrogens. Continuing research suggests that these herbs do not always increase a woman's estrogen. Herbs with plant hormones do not behave like hormone drugs. Some studies suggest that phytoestrogens can decrease the risk of cancer, presumably by competing with estrogen, which can cause cancer.

Some herbal remedies for menopause contain the plant hormone beta-sitosterol, and the herbs they contain only act like estrogen in women whose estrogen is unusually low. Examples of herbs containing some amount, large or small, of beta-sitosterol are dong quai, licorice, ginseng, saw palmetto, calendula, St. John's wort, and red clover. Others containing phytoestrogens, such as alfalfa, showed both estrogenic and anti-estrogenic effects in experiments, though these animal experiments from the 1960s are, in my opinion, always suspect. Having said that, this maybe-yes-maybe-no test result is in keeping with other plants that, like alfalfa, contain both isoflavones and coumestrol.

The menopausal herb chasteberry *(Vitex agnus-castus)* is native to Greek islands and sacred to the goddess Hera, mythological protectress of married women and mothers. This herb affects the pituitary gland in the brain, with effects on luteinizing hormone, follicle-stimulating hormone, and prolactin. Herbalists commonly speak of chasteberry as promoting progesterone. While it appears that way, this action is unproven. A more exact description is that chasteberry promotes the rebalancing of hormonal signals between the brain and ovaries. In turn, this action helps normalize progesterone and estrogen levels. Another profertility fruit in mythology of the Mediterranean basin is the pomegranate, which, like the date palm, contains some estrone.

Herbs that contain diosgenin, sarsapogenin, or related compounds include wild yam *(Dioscorea villosa)*, blue cohosh *(Caulophyllum thalictroides)*, fenugreek *(Trigonella foenum-graecum)*, wild sarsaparilla *(Smilax* species), and the reliable women's remedy, bethroot *(Trillium* species), which is now endangered by overharvesting.

Some doctors warn women about the dangers of using herbs that have hormonal effects. Perhaps they have not read the research suggesting the protective benefits of plant estrogens, even on estrogen-sensitive growths. A far greater source of concern for all of us is the widespread presence of human-made compounds known to have harmful estrogenic effects, especially in breast and other reproductive tissues. For instance, in Israel, the rate of breast cancer dropped significantly after the use of DDT was banned. This is not proof that all chemicals are evil or that all hormonal herbs are harmless. It simply means that additional factors require study, and that doctors shouldn't be so quick to label an herb as unsafe until they know the plant's full range of uses and effects, as any good herbalist should.

Natural Hormone Replacement
or HRT: Your Decision

Physicians are not the only people jumping to false conclusions about estrogenic herbs. There is a booming market of herbal products providing natural progesterone "from herbs." Some products may have pronounced effects on a woman's health when used as directed, some may be made with extracts of wild yam, and some may be made with the best intentions of providing women with alternatives to synthetic hormones. But let's be clear: No amount of external creams or ingested herbal products from these whole plants have been shown to cause an increase in a woman's progesterone. The whole herbs and genuinely natural products made from them have many other healing attributes for women in menopause; increasing sex hormone levels is not one of them. These herbal steroids are not converted *naturally* into progesterone in our metabolism but in the lab. If a company claims that a month's worth of cream containing wild yam extract (a 2-ounce jar) delivers 900 milligrams of "natural progesterone," it cannot have made the cream without doctoring the herbal diosgenin in a laboratory. Some companies simply use wild yam extracts and add animal progesterone, usually from "affordable raw materials." This is the polite phrase for pregnant mare's urine—the same ingredient that drug companies make into Premarin.

There is no agreement on the optimal type of drug regime or duration of monitoring by physicians. It is agreed that HRT's side effects are in proportion to the strength of the dose and the length of time on it. There is no consensus on adding progesterones to ERT, prescribed to women who have undergone removal of the uterus. They are the usual population given ERT because there is no risk of cancer of the uterine lining. Can cancer be induced elsewhere if the hormones induce it in tissues such as the uterine lining? No one can say.

Progesterone, like estrogen, may lower incidence of bone loss, but the route of administration and the long-term effects of HRT for this effect are still debated. The use of patches or creams releases hormones directly into the bloodstream, so the risks of high blood levels of estrogen (emboli, high blood pressure) may apply. Vaginal creams release hormones into the bloodstream as well, but in very small amounts. If the HRT is administered orally (pills), the liver can process the hormones like any drug or substance taken by mouth. But this is associated with a two to three times higher risk of gallbladder disease, perhaps to the point of gallstones, pain, poor fat metabolism, and surgery.

As with gallbladder problems, there is an uncertain relationship between estrogen levels and osteoporosis—the fear of which is a big reason doctors push HRT on women. Though a real condition, only one-quarter of postmenopausal women develop osteoporosis in the ten to twenty years *after* menopause, and even then it is linked with much more than low estrogen levels. As for osteoporosis tests, they have their problems as well. They are expensive and so are less likely to be done in a consistent way. They may also be misleading. One examination will measure the forearm's bone density, but this says little about a woman's weight-bearing vertebrae or hip. If another costly test measures the spine and hips, it is still unclear how much bone loss in one location leads to a site of fracture. If there are no signs or symptoms of osteoporosis in a young to middle-aged woman, the tests for predicting it may be especially inconclusive. A CT ("cat") Scan has the same drawbacks but with a higher radiation dose. If bone tests are helpful because of personal or family history, ask your health-care provider to suggest the best type for you.

Women with or without hot flashes can have the same circulating amount of estrogen, so HRT is no guarantee of avoiding hot flashes. And why should women avoid them, unless they are debilitating? Moreover, this symptom may recur on withdrawal from HRT, which a woman may choose to do every three to six months. This allows a woman to reassess whether natural remedies have helped her make any health progress. Further, a woman and her physician can check the need for renewing a prescription or lowering the dosage. Vaginal estrogen creams are better when used briefly, if at all. The natural approach for the symptom of vaginal thinning is often as reliable, especially for sensitive women. It involves Kegel exercises, love and sex, or natural lubricants with a local effect of increasing tissue levels of estrogen. An example is the wild yam cream described elsewhere.

Most women find HRT superfluous even if they have not been taking perfect care of their health. That is not to say that HRT is always superfluous. Natural therapists will honor the healing value of any approach, including HRT, if it is truly healing in the context of a woman's life. Some women are helped by HRT. We all deserve respect for our health choices, without judgment from "healers" or ourselves. I just ask women and their health-care providers to know the pros and cons. To be sure, check the literature. There are references in the bibliography at the end of this book. Talk with other women. Don't take my word for any of this. Don't take the word of a drug representative. Or a doctor. Or an herbalist. And certainly not a manufacturer of products. Decide for yourself about your need for HRT, from your own place of power and free choice.

Premature Menopause

Premature menopause is defined as a sudden or unhealthy drop in estrogen, after puberty but before the range of normal menopause (thirty-six to sixty-five, usually fifty or fifty-one). In some cultures the mid- to late thirties are not considered an unhealthy age for menopause. The first irregular cycles and hot flashes at this age do not automatically mean there is a health problem. There may be simple causes, remedied naturally at this stage. If self-care and using herbs don't resolve a woman's symptoms in three months or so, it may help to see a health professional. The ovaries may not ovulate every month and some hormonal changes may be felt long before menopause. Premature menopause is something else. If a woman enters menopause before she has matured into it naturally, the cause may be some form of ill health. This is often linked to smoking, chemotherapy, radiation, and, of course, surgical removal of reproductive organs at any age.

Conventional medicine believes that leaving in the ovaries allows a "natural" menopause, but an estimated half of the women who have undergone removal of the uterus but not the ovaries still lose some or all ovarian function. Why do ovaries stop functioning sooner than expected when not connected to a uterus? Because women react differently to traumas, including surgery, and we are not an assembly of separately moving parts. Still, sometimes this surgical choice is a woman's best chance for health. Though most hysterectomies are now considered to have been unnecessary, the imbalances leading to them are abundant on our planet. Many surgeries, such as oophorectomy (removal of ovaries) in DES daughters, are a cause of premature menopause unknown in past centuries. It has been estimated that in the 1980s, 12 million women in the United States were surgically initiated into menopause. Certainly, there are health risks as we grow older, but no one body organ is the "cause" of our most feared, most complex health problems. Our parts are built up from DNA protein blueprints found in every cell, and that does not change the minute we are done bearing children. Our body parts are not meant to be surgically removed or drugged into obedience just because someone else says we won't be needing them now. When reproductive organs hurt, this pain may be a difficult signpost to have, but it is the body's most effective way to get our attention. We may choose surgery or medication, but these are not the only responses to body signals.

In health, the body works at *not* producing estrogenic hormones around menopause, except in smaller amounts. We are asking for trouble when we feed women a dose of hormones to avoid health problems. How can we ask why breast cancer, unexplainable endometriosis, and gynecological disease is on the rise, despite all the advances we have seen in medicine? HRT is not the cause of all these ills, but our culture's lack of consciousness with our use of technology is partly responsible.

The median age for women going through a surgical menopause is forty-one, usually because of fibroids (more or less half these women), or premature menopause due to severe illness, such as cancer. One-third of Western women over age fifty at the time of this writing are still having hysterectomies—having their "organs of hysteria" removed. There are wildly different rates for this in the United States, the statistics showing two differences: by regions and by ethnicity, with different rates for African American, Latina, and Native American women and Caucasian women. Fibroids are a poor reason for a hysterectomy because more conservative options exist. Women surgeons have pioneered the use of myomectomies (just removing the fibroid, not the womb), and fibroids often shrink at menopause when estrogen levels drop naturally. At any age, women with fibroids can change the foods that affect this condition and use reproductive tonics with astringent herbs to shrink the fibroids faster while improving their general health.

Women should keep their wombs. An exception in my opinion may be when there is a fast-growing fibroid for which natural therapies may not be the first treatment choice. The womb is not just for carrying a pregnancy to term. This cauldron of creative life is important all through life. If a woman's womb bothers her, she might question if she is bothering it, asking herself what the messages of her womb convey, instead of removing the organ that is signaling to her so insistently. There are no pat answers, just worthwhile questions.

If life-threatening, noncancerous conditions are the reason for surgical menopause, especially in women of a young age, the benefits of HRT may outweigh the side effects. Even in such a case, all women starting HRT between twenty-six and thirty-six do not report good results. Some young women without ovaries love HRT, but others refuse to stay on hormones because of side effects and poor quality of life. In my experience, the health of these women who will not take HRT will improve with natural health-care techniques, including nutrition and herbs. All of the herbal formulas and recommendations in this book may be tried by women thrust prematurely into menopause. Listen to yourself first and health-care providers afterward—but do keep in contact with a health professional you trust.

Coming Off HRT Safely

Many women already know they want to stop taking HRT and try herbs. If you have symptoms or just feel unwell on hormones, wean off them slowly. Several dosage combinations exist. What was standard ten years ago is considered barbarically high within some medical circles today. One of the more common low doses of conjugated estrogen (for example, Premarin) prescribed is 0.3 milligram. The middle dose is 0.625 milligram and the higher dose is 1.25 milligrams per day. For estradiol (for example, Estrace), the dose ranges from 0.5 milligram up to 1.0 milligram per day. These are taken from days 1 through 25; then 2.5 to 10 milligrams of progestin are taken for at least seven to ten days; this is repeated for three to six months. Unless your health-care provider has some outstanding reason for keeping you at the same dose, you probably can use those three to six months to slowly reduce your dosage to a lower level. At that time, women are encouraged to wean off and reassess whether they feel better without the HRT, even if they have a little bit of rebound hot flashes.

If you need to continue longer on HRT at any dose, you can start using the following herbs at the same time. Follow this stair-step, safe, and slow plan over the next three to six months. It may seem as if it goes on forever. But it usually is better for our bodies to follow a consistent, predictable routine when we are making major changes. If you want to go faster than this, I cannot reach out of the pages and stop you. The deciding factor is how well you are. The first step is to take "First Freedom" extract or tea, described below, for at least four weeks along with your regular dose of HRT on the regular cycle. This allows the body to recognize and get accustomed to metabolizing the milder hormone-balancing herbs before starting to slowly wean off the hormones.

If women are using a patch (for example, Estraderm) instead of taking oral medication, the dose is 0.05 milligram to 0.1 milligram every three to four days. This delivery of the drug (estrogen) is through the skin. Our bodies were designed to pass everything, especially hormones, through the liver. Regardless, the same herbs below can be used. Lower dose patches can be prescribed over time, or women can achieve similar results themselves. During the first month, take the herbs along with regular use and replacement of the patch. During the next phase wait an extra day before replacing the patch. Each time you feel ready to withstand any rebound symptoms, add another day before replacing the patch. Stretch this out as slowly as it is comfortable or manageable. You can speed up the process according to your own preference. Always see a supportive health-care provider if this brings up problems. The two of you may easily identify the problems so they can be handled simply, or additional care may be required.

Herbal Medicine

FIRST FREEDOM

Extracts	Botanical Names	Actions
4 oz. black cohosh root	*Cimicifuga racemosa*	Estrogenic relaxing tonic
3 oz. fennel seed	*Foeniculum vulgare*	Limits bloating and gas
3 oz. red clover flower	*Trifolium pratense*	Mild estrogenic lymphatic and nerve tonic

Ten ounces will last thirty days. Combine these herbal extracts. Take 1 teaspoon in 1 cup water twice a day, morning and evening.

FIRST FREEDOM TEA

Dried Herbs	Botanical Names	Actions
7 oz. black cohosh root	*Cimicifuga racemosa*	Estrogenic relaxing tonic
4 oz. fennel seed	*Foeniculum vulgare*	Limits bloating and gas
4 oz. red clover flower	*Trifolium pratense*	Mild estrogenic lymphatic and nerve tonic

Fifteen ounces will last thirty days. Add 1/2 ounce of the mixture to 3 1/2 cups of boiling water in a teapot or container with a well-fitting lid. Let stand for twenty minutes before straining. Drink 1 cup hot or cold three times a day.

During the second month on both herbs and regular HRT dose, reduce the dose of HRT by one-quarter (or less if you are very sensitive). Lowering the dose of the powerful hormones may result in a few symptoms. You can minimize symptoms by taking "Lion Tamer" instead of "First Freedom." Every time the HRT is reduced, the herb formula changes. This is usually done in one-month stages. Your body will appreciate the change of herbal flavors and benefits. You can make every stage last for two months if there is a reason to be extra-cautious. These combinations, when taken as directed, are safe enough for most women to take as often as they need in order to feel well. The herbs are far more mild than the drug regime, so do not be afraid to take frequent sips of tea all day or droppers of extracts every ten minutes until you get good results.

Just for comparison, the birth control pill is 2,500 micrograms DES equivalents, postmenopausal HRT is 500 micrograms DES equivalents, and the most potent plant estrogen, coumestrol, in the form of 20 grams dry-weight soybeans (sprouted), is 0.5 microgram. This is not as weak as it looks on paper or in lab tests because many natural plant hormones can be converted over time to more active forms during metabolism. Just know vegetable hormones are not as druglike in their effects as pharmaceutical HRT.

❦————————————LION TAMER————————————❦

Extracts	Botanical Names	Actions
3 oz. dong quai root	*Angelica sinensis*	Estrogenic circulatory and immune tonic
1 oz. licorice root	*Glycyrrhiza glabra*	Anti-inflammatory; adrenal and antiviral digestive aid
1 oz. peppermint leaf	*Mentha piperita*	Reduces bloating and gas
1 oz. motherwort herb	*Leonurus cardiaca*	Reduces hot flashes; aids liver metabolism
1 oz. Siberian ginseng root	*Eleutherococcus senticosus*	Improves stress and immune response

Ten ounces will last thirty days. Combine these herbal extracts. Take 1 teaspoon in 1 cup water twice a day, morning and evening.

Dried Herbs	Botanical Names	Actions
6 oz. dong quai root	*Angelica sinensis*	Estrogenic circulatory and immune tonic
3 oz. Siberian ginseng root	*Eleutherococcus senticosus*	Improves stress and immune response
2 oz. licorice root	*Glycyrrhiza glabra*	Anti-inflammatory; adrenal and antiviral digestive aid
2 oz. peppermint leaf	*Mentha piperita*	Reduces bloating and gas
1 oz. motherwort herb	*Leonurus cardiaca*	Reduces hot flashes; aids liver metabolism

Fifteen ounces will last 30 days. Add 1/2 ounce of the mixture to 3 1/2 cups of boiling water in a teapot or container with a well-fitting lid. Let stand for fifteen minutes before straining. Drink 1 cup hot or cold three times a day. If you prefer, sip tea throughout the day or drink two larger glasses twice a day, but make sure you drink 3 cups a day.

In the third month, if all is going well and you want to continue the process, reduce HRT by another one-quarter (to one-half the original dose). If you experience severe symptoms, go back to the last HRT dose that was comfortable and continue the herbs for an extra month or more, until you feel ready to try reducing the dose again. If you are very sensitive, only reduce by one-quarter at this stage, to three-quarters of the normal dose. During this month, take "Smooth Sailing."

Extracts	Botanical Names	Actions
2 oz. chasteberry seed	*Vitex agnus-castus*	Promotes progesterene; reduces hot flashes
2 oz. skullcap herb	*Scutellaria laterifolia*	Relaxing nerve tonic
2 oz. Jamaican sarsaparilla root	*Smilax ornata*	Hormonal balancing; lymphatic and immune tonic
2 oz. dandelion root	*Taraxacum officinale*	Provides minerals; aids liver metabolism
2 oz. fennel seed	*Foeniculum vulgare*	Reduces bloating and gas

Ten ounces will last thirty days. Combine these herbal extracts. Take 1 teaspoon in 1 cup water, diluted juice, or herb tea in the morning and evening.

Dried Herbs	Botanical Names	Actions
4 oz. chasteberry seed	*Vitex agnus-castus*	Promotes progesterene; reduces hot flashes
3 oz. skullcap herb	*Scutellaria laterifolia*	Relaxing nerve tonic
3 oz. Jamaican sarsaparilla root	*Smilax ornata*	Hormonal balancing; lymphatic and immune tonic
3 oz. dandelion root	*Taraxacum officinale*	Provides minerals; aids liver metabolism
2 oz. fennel seed	*Foeniculum vulgare*	Reduces bloating and gas

Fifteen ounces will last thirty days. Add 1/2 ounce of the mixture to 3 1/2 cups of boiling water in a teapot or container with a well-fitting lid. Let stand for fifteen minutes before straining. Drink 1 cup hot or cold three times a day.

During the fourth month, drop from half dose down to one-quarter dose and go back on "First Freedom." Once you are on a quarter dose or less, the process goes a little faster. If you are sensitive or like to take the slower method just in case, take a fifth month to drop another one-eighth off the dose and go back on "Lion Tamer." If you need to take a sixth month until you are taking one-eighth of your original dose, also take "Smooth Sailing."

You may at any time go back up to the last dose of HRT and herbs that felt comfortable through the month. If this occurs more than once, pay attention to your nutrition, make sure you have outlets for stress like exercise, and consider other factors. Give yourself time. And let your health-care provider know what you are doing!

Finally, when you are taking only one-quarter or one-eighth of your original HRT dose, plus the herbs, take the HRT every other day for that whole cycle. In the next cycle, take the same small dose every third day. You will know you are ready for another dose reduction when you can honestly feel that your health signs are stable as the drugs are slowly withdrawn. In the next cycle after that, take the hormones every four days. Then, only take the same small dose (one-quarter or one-eighth for the very sensitive) once a week for another cycle. When you are taking the hormones only once a week, try dropping them all together. Stay on the herb combination you are taking at that time.

The whole process of weaning off may be complete in one month or ten, but normally it will not take longer than a full year. If it does because of other medication or chronic health issues, you may require more time or more guidance from your health-care provider.

Expecting miracles is a two-sided coin. You may have quick, terrific results, or you may feel disappointed if your symptoms are still hanging around. Herbs may or may not make your biggest symptoms disappear overnight like magic. Share experiences with other women, but try to avoid comparing yourself with them. Look instead for longer periods of time without bad hot flashes, a few better nights of sleep in a week, or other markers you may notice.

Remember, the body in health likes rhythm. HRT is made up of powerful chemicals. You may choose to drop your dosage at a faster rate if you have a supportive health-care provider, but whatever you do, be consistent. Quick drops in estrogen cause drops in calcium mineralization of the bone—the biggest reason for slow withdrawal. Please don't do as many women tell me they have done, which is to just get fed up and throw the prescription away all at once. Some women are fine when they do this, and it is one choice among many. Please know going off HRT all at once may be easy for one woman and horrible for another. It boils down to knowing oneself.

When this gradual dose reduction is complete, switch to the following new and simple formula for one more month.

🌿 ———————— FINAL FREEDOM ———————— 🌿

Extracts	Botanical Names	Actions
2 oz. rosehips	*Rosa canina*	Circulatory, nutritive, cooling tonic
2 oz. fennel seeds	*Foeniculum vulgare*	Estrogenic digestive aid
6 oz. red clover flower	*Trifolium pratense*	Mild estrogenic lymphatic and nerve tonic

Ten ounces will last thirty days. Combine these herbal extracts. Take 1 teaspoon in 1 cup water, diluted juice, or herb tea in the morning and evening.

🌿 ———————— FINAL FREEDOM TEA ———————— 🌿

Extracts	Botanical Names	Actions
4 oz. rosehips	*Rosa canina*	Circulatory, nutritive, cooling tonic
4 oz. fennel seeds	*Foeniculum vulgare*	Estrogenic digestive aid
7 oz. red clover flower	*Trifolium pratense*	Mild estrogenic lymphatic and nerve tonic

Fifteen ounces will last thirty days. Add 1/2 ounce of the mixture to 3 1/2 cups of boiling water in a teapot or container with a well-fitting lid. Let stand for fifteen minutes before straining. Drink 1 cup hot or cold three times a day.

Because you are taking herbs and not hormone stimulants as you slowly decrease estrogen, the relative drop in estrogen will mean that sometimes there is no buildup of the uterine lining. For that reason, if you have a uterus and if you have been used to having a monthly release of blood, don't worry when it skips and ends. If you are concerned about this, consult with a trusted, supportive health-care provider. It is also always wise to continue regular checkups for general wellness and your own particular health concerns.

Chapter 4

POSTMENOPAUSE

In his novel *Intruders in the Dust*, William Faulkner writes that if one needs an impossible task accomplished, a wrong righted, or a noble effort performed with grace and skill, forget elected officials, venerated city fathers, or even energetic youths—ask an old woman. There is profound truth in this observation. Vital older women have great life wisdom and know how to get things done.

After menopause, many women find themselves moving out of an intense phase of child rearing and career building to pursue new passions and adventures. For some, it brings the freedom to accomplish deep personal transformation. But for many women, this vital third of life brings critical challenges, particularly in the areas of health and financial security. Many senior women fear retirement because they lack sufficient income to meet their basic needs. Loss of a life partner and distance from family members add to the emotional and survival issues faced by older women.

Whatever your personal circumstances, your postmenopausal years offer you a new opportunity to change how you care for yourself, to strengthen body, mind, and spirit, to face challenges that arise, as well as to energize you to pursue new interests. Keeping active and fit, eating wisely, and supporting your well-being with herbs and other natural therapies can help minimize potential health threats and maintain and renew your zest for life. Buoyed by new energy and courage, you can continue to do the impossible.

This chapter discusses herbal and other natural remedies for some of the most common health conditions affecting postmenopausal women. Teas are generally more beneficial than extracts in the postmenopausal period, especially if you are taking multiple medications for health problems, because they are more water soluble and safer. They also help prevent dehydration in older women who do not drink enough liquids or who suffer from diabetes or illnesses accompanied by diarrhea or vomiting. When dehydration is not a problem, herbal extract combinations can give quick relief.

The following herbal mixtures are formulated so you can safely use the faster-acting extracts along with the milder teas without fear of overdosing. The teas are effective by themselves for long-standing conditions and may be a more affordable option.

Arthritis

Arthritis is an inflammation where two bones meet in a joint. Painful joints are more than a "mechanical" annoyance: They are especially hard to cope with when the hands are affected or when pain in the knees and hips makes exercise difficult to enjoy. Arthritis is linked to insomnia, stress, other physical changes, and depression. Depression is commonly undiagnosed when it is combined with arthritis.

There are two main types of arthritis: "wear-and-tear arthritis," or osteoarthritis, and an autoimmune type called "rheumatoid arthritis." Osteoarthritis, associated with years of repeated physical movement that wears some joints out faster than others, usually affects joints in the hips, shoulders, fingers, and neck. In osteoarthritis, there is a loss of the glassy-smooth cartilage where two bones meet, so the bones rub against each other. The body responds by making the whole area stiff, swollen, red, and sore in the hope it will be rested instead of stressed further. While injury or sports may worsen the condition, so will inactivity: Surrounding muscles contract, further drawing the bones close up against each other. When they rub, the friction causes more heat and more friction. Damp weather also causes muscle contraction and can worsen the condition, as can stress, which may be reflected in unconscious tension placed on joints and other vulnerable spots in the body. The following formulas therefore contain herbs that relax muscle tension.

Rheumatoid arthritis usually starts as an illness accompanied by fevers and joint pain that moves around the body or comes and goes. Because this form of arthritis isn't due to wear and tear but is in the bloodstream, it may hit non-weight-bearing joints and the same joints on both sides of the body (both elbows, both thumbs, and so forth). It may coexist with other autoimmune conditions.

The cause of rheumatoid arthritis is debated, but it is apparently an autoimmune disorder. Immune cells consider the cells lining the joints to be foreign invaders, so they attack them, resulting in inflammation, pain, and stiffness. Like all autoimmune conditions, rheumatoid arthritis is complex enough for a woman to seek professional health care, but the recommendations below may improve it, and they are not likely to make it worse.

A woman can have both types of arthritis because autoimmune destruction of a joint can lead to wear and tear. Though family history may be associated with these diseases, you don't automatically inherit them just because a parent or grandparent has joint problems. Diagnosis in both cases is confirmed by X-rays and blood tests.

If you have arthritis or think you are a candidate for it, you especially need to eat wisely, keep fit, and carry body fat lightly. The ten extra pounds or so that women usually gain after menopause are protective provided they are composed of a mixture of muscle and dense bone developed from exercising and a little cushioning of fat under the skin. The fat cells help maintain our internal balance of estrogen as well as protect us in case we take a tumble. Exercise additionally helps by improving coordination even when joints are stiff and achey. Stretching or enjoying yoga designed for elders can safely return freedom of movement to your body.

Neck stiffness caused by arthritis can lead to frequent headaches, but you should avoid the temptation to regularly take aspirin or painkillers for them or for joint pain. Frequent use can eventually damage the stomach lining, reduce liver cell function, and worsen ringing in your ears, not to mention cause other known or possible side effects. The natural salicylates found in willow and meadowsweet are not concentrated enough for some headaches, but they can help reduce their severity or prevent future headaches.

Although simple techniques like dietary changes, exercise, and herbal preparations may not reverse changes to bone tissue, they can mitigate arthritic symptoms. The following herbal formulas can help clear the body of inflmmatory "junk" that triggers flare-ups. Because pain and other body changes related to arthritis may well bring on depression, some of the herbs traditionally used for arthritic pain, swelling, and stiffness are also nutritive, relaxing yet mood lifting, and sometimes anti-inflammatory.

Herbal Medicine

❦ ───────────────── WILLOW GRACE ───────────────── ❦

Extracts	Botanical Names	Actions
4 oz. willow bark	*Salix alba*	Reduces inflammation, pain
2 oz. St. John's wort herb	*Hypericum perforatum*	Antidepressant; repairs nerves; strengthens immunity
2 oz. alfalfa leaf	*Medicago sativa*	Nutritive, antiarthritic; provides minerals
2 oz. black cohosh root	*Cimicifuga racemosa*	Antiarthritic; relaxes nerves; hormonal tonic

Ten ounces will last thirty days. Combine these herbal extracts. Take 1 teaspoon in 1 cup water, juice, or any herb tea in the morning and evening.

Dried Herbs	Botanical Names	Actions
5 oz. willow bark	*Salix alba*	Reduces inflammation; improves elimination through kidneys
3 oz. black cohosh root	*Cimicifuga racemosa*	Antiarthritic; relaxes nerves; supports hormonal balance
3 oz. meadowsweet herb	*Filipendula ulmaria*	Anti-inflammatory; heals stomach lining; for taste
2 oz. St. John's wort herb	*Hypericum perforatum*	Antidepressant; repairs nerves; strengthens immunity
1 oz. alfalfa leaf	*Medicago sativa*	Nutritive, antiarthritic; provides minerals
1 oz. burdock root	*Arctium lappa*	Nutritive, antiarthritic; reduces sugar craving

Fifteen ounces will last thirty days. Add 1/2 ounce of the mixture to 3 1/2 cups of boiling water in a teapot or container with a well-fitting lid. Let stand for fifteen minutes before straining. Drink 1 cup hot or cold three times a day. If you prefer, sip tea all day or drink two large glasses twice a day, making sure you drink 3 cups a day.

Nutrition

Wise Food Choices
- Eat steamed dark green vegetables at least twice a week, but avoid spinach, rhubarb, and other oxalate-containing vegetables and fruits.
- Limit or avoid alcohol, as it is a depressant and contributes to some women's arthritis. If you want a glass of wine at dinner to help digestion or sleep, avoid red wine because red grape products worsen arthritis. For this reason, also avoid red grapes, red wine vinegar, and purple grape juice.
- Limit or avoid coffee (decaffeinated or regular), dairy products (from cows, especially milk, cheese, and butter), potatoes, tomatoes, eggplants, cayenne pepper, black pepper, and bell or green peppers.

In Addition
- Add 10 drops of lavender essential oil to a comfortably hot bath; swish the water to disperse the oil. Light a candle in a safe place, close the door, and

soak your bones, smoothing the lavender water into your skin. Skip the soap tonight; relax for at least twenty minutes. If you've had an active day, let out the water and start a new bath as many times as you wish, until your toes and fingers "prune." Finish with a lukewarm or cool shower, and move slowly: the heat dilates blood vessels, causing some sensitive women to feel dizzy if they stand or exit the tub too quickly. If you have high blood pressure, avoid extremes of temperature and use common sense.

- To relieve pain in hands and wrists, find a salad bowl or a large, shallow container that you can easily fit your hands into. In this bowl, stir a table-spoon of dried yellow mustard powder and a little warm water into a paste. Keep adding comfortably hot water, about 4 cups (1 quart), squishing out lumps as you turn the paste into a thin, watery broth. Reserve some of the liquid; then place your hands in the bowl of hot mustard water and soak them for ten to twenty minutes, occasionally adding in a little more mustard powder broth or hot water to keep hand bath comfortably hot when it cools down. After the first five minutes, begin to open and close your fists, mas-saging painful knuckles and joints, until swelling and stiffness have lessened and movement is easier. Rinse with lukewarm, plain water and pat (do not rub) dry. Your hands should tingle. You can repeat the treatment daily for a week or until internal remedies begin to make it less necessary. Do not use with open cuts, burns, or skin rashes; mustard can be irritating.

- You can purchase or make a cayenne ointment and massage it into larger areas, such as the hips, knees, and lower back. Alternatively, massage the area for ten minutes or more with 1 ounce almond oil and 1/4 ounce essential oil of wintergreen. Methyl salicylate, commonly available at drugstores, is not as nice smelling but may be effective also.

- What about DMSO? This anti-inflammatory chemical (dimethyl sulfoxide) may be pain relieving, but its use is controversial. For some, it is a lifesaver; for others, it may stop being effective or may have side effects. It smells like garlic, which you may consider a disadvantage. I do not have enough expe-rience with DMSO over several years to form a conclusion about its efficacy.

- Therapeutic sweats are a traditional way to rejuvenate a tired body. Contact health spas or saunas in your local area; ask personnel for information about cautions and benefits of steam rooms or hot tubs.

- Any amount of exercise helps, no matter how little you think you can do. Especially healing are activities involving slow movement: tai chi, stretching, swimming, yoga, and dance. Be sure to let the class instructor know your interest, level of fitness, and special concerns. Remember that unaccustomed new movements may work muscles you have forgotten about and cause soreness, but if you do not feel better soon, find a more receptive teacher; many are trained in older women's fitness.

- Try the following visualization. Sit or stand, feet flat on the floor, weight distributed evenly. Imagine yourself just as you are. Pressing your shoulders back and dropping them down, breathe in and out evenly and slowly. See your bones as levers. Imagine that when they move they are pulling muscles. For five or ten minutes, picture your muscles smoothly and comfortably performing the movements you make each day. Visualize your movements as realistically as you can. Perhaps you see yourself picking something up from the floor, reaching up to close a window. If you wince when you imagine any movement, take a slow breath, count to ten, and then imagine it again in slow motion, visualizing it as effortless movement, even if it is a different reach or stretch. Straighten your spine to lengthen it a few inches while you continue to breathe. Stretch your hands out and make fists; then relax them. Allow your vision to clear so you can know the image of the body you already have within yourself waiting to be realized. If you are sitting, rise as slowly as you can, concentrating only on feeling the subtle changes you have already begun to visualize in your mind.

Changing Nutritional Needs

You may find that you can't eat salads anymore without suffering from indigestion. Indigestion from lettuce and other "health" foods may be traced to low levels of stomach acid, which needs to be produced in sufficient quantity to break down roughage and extract vitamins and minerals from the indigestible cellulose of plant foods. But why do many older women have low stomach acid? Loading up on calcium carbonate and chalky dolomite supplements for ten or fifteen years is one possibility; daily consumption of calcium-rich antacid tablets is another.

Nevertheless, not all women who experience indigestion take calcium supplements, so every case can't be the fault of supplements alone. In fact, efficient digestion gradually decreases with aging. But digestive problems have as much to do with the chemically treated factory-farm produce generally available in stores.

One way to improve nutrition as you age is to lightly steam fresh vegetables to make them more digestible, switch to other staples like whole grains, and rekindle a strong digestive metabolism with nutritive herbs and vegetables. These plants, called "bitters," also help stabilize blood sugar by stimulating the proteins and sugars stored in the pancreas, liver, and blood. For this reason they can help women with diabetes; in addition, they help women with low blood sugar control their cravings for refined sugar. Therefore, they are recommended to any woman with a diabetic condition. Because diabetes can worsen with age or multiple medication, every healthful technique you can use to help you avoid increasing the necessary dose of oral hypoglycemics—like using nutritive herbs—is worth practicing. For insulin-dependent diabetes, close monitoring of blood sugar changes and checking with your physician are always recommended.

Changing nutritional needs and changing digestion may include constipation. This is not a failure of your body; rather, it may be your body's healthy signal that you must eat differently now or else! You can resolve the problem most simply by drinking more fluids. For some women, though, it is hard to force down extra water or liquids. Since the 1930s the common wisdom was to drink six to eight glasses of water a day. Yet some women are going to feel inadequate, even guilty, if they can't manage this because of urinary frequency. Eating more soups and fewer animal proteins is one way to ease the burden on digestion. The digestive tea included below is not specific to constipation, but the herbs it contains will get the old digestive motors up and running and stimulate the liver to regulate nutrient balance and bowel function. Avoid regular use of herbal laxatives that irritate the colon *(senna* and *cascara sagrada)*. These are particularly bad if you are trying to lose weight because emptying the colon is not the same as burning off unwanted fat, and they may provoke diarrhea, pain, and other symptoms. The occasional use of laxatives to relieve constipation for one or two nights at a time can be helpful, but because they work by irritating your colon's nerve endings, don't use them unless they're really needed.

A third area of concern is bloating and gas. The problem is that food may not digest as well and create more "bad" bacteria in your stomach; then the bacteria throw a party and then leave you to deal with the consequences—more gas. Whether particular foods, genetic predisposition, or something as yet unclear to us is responsible, the answer is to eat differently. As with the previous two health concerns, blood sugar and constipation, use bitter salad vegetables (such as endive and chicory) and whole foods to stimulate peristalsis for normal bowel movement and reverse a tendency to constipation, combined with gas-reducing aromatic herbs such as fennel seeds, thyme, rosemary, or the Mexican herb epazote, cooked with beans to reduce flatulence. In addition to eating bitter salad vegetables, avoid foods that cause gas and bloating and use volatile oil-containing herbs to clear out the bulk of the bad bacteria. These tend to be herbs that taste good, add spice to dishes, and sweeten the breath—for example, cinnamon, sage, and other favorite culinary herbs. You can take the following extract or tea after heavy meals to settle digestive upsets, clear intestinal gas, and nourish the body parts that nourish you.

Herbal Medicine

Extracts	Botanical Names	Actions
1 oz. peppermint leaf	*Mentha piperita*	Antiseptic; kills bad bacteria; reduces gas
1 oz. lemon balm leaf	*Melissa officinalis*	Lifts spirits; reduces bloating; antiviral
1 oz. chamomile flower	*Matricaria recutita*	Soothes nerves; quiets intestinal spasms
1 oz. yellow dock root	*Rumex crispus*	Bitter; supports liver's metabolism of fats; contains iron
1 oz. fennel seed	*Foeniculum vulgare*	For taste; harmonizes herbs

Five ounces will last for ten days of regular use, or longer if used occasionally. Combine these extracts. Take 1 to 2 teaspoons diluted in 1 cup water after or between meals, as needed, up to three times a day. If you are allergic to chrysanthemum flowers or chamomile itself, leave them out.

————————— IN MINT CONDITION TEA —————————

Dried Herbs	Botanical Names	Actions
1 oz. peppermint leaf	*Mentha piperita*	Antiseptic; kills bad bacteria; reduces gas
1 oz. lemon balm leaf	*Melissa officinalis*	Lifts spirits; reduces bloating; antiviral
1 oz. chamomile flower	*Matricaria recutita*	Soothes nerves; quiets intestinal spasms
1 oz. yellow dock root	*Rumex crispus*	Bitter; supports liver's metabolism of fats; contains iron
1 oz. fennel seed	*Foeniculum vulgare*	For taste; harmonizes herbs

Five ounces will last for five to ten days of regular use, or longer if used occasionally. For quick relief, add 1 ounce of the combination to 2 to 3 cups boiling water in a teapot with a well-fitting lid or other covered container. Let sit fifteen minutes; strain and drink 1/2 cup before each meal and 1/2 cup afterward up to four times a day for five days. For occasional need or for use as an enjoyable digestive beverage, add 1 to 2 teaspoons of this mixture to 1 cup boiling water and leave covered for ten to fifteen minutes; then strain and drink as desired. Best after or between meals, as needed, up to three times each day. If you are allergic to chrysanthemum flowers or chamomile itself, leave them out.

A note about weight gain: It is usual, no matter how little you eat, to experience some weight gain postmenopausally. Over time, gravity pulls us into a charming pear shape and our thighs thicken no matter how much we exercise. For many women, the problem with this change isn't the weight per se; it's the rapid weight gain in fat that makes us feel bad—both because of how our bodies feel and because we are somehow not conforming to our culture's standard, preferred image of health and attractiveness.

The best way to deal with weight gain is twofold: to exercise daily or weekly over the months and years, so that the weight is added in the form of dense bone, muscle, and only a little extra fat; and to be your own advocate for your health and self-image. To do so, you will need to evaluate your own needs and reality and dismiss other people's prejudices. Do you need to lose some weight to lessen the strain on your heart or arthritic bones? Or is this the time to loosen up about your waistline and accept yourself as you are? Only you can decide. Beware of easy, feel-good answers that are not your truth. It is not "feminist" to be unhealthy and risk a heart attack just because the dominant society sells products using male-oriented sexual imagery. Remaining overweight as a protest against society or as protection against sexual advances does not give us equal rights; only self-knowledge and free choice can do that, whatever the scales say. Be wary of herb products or diets promising quick results. Only through slow, careful care—exercise and proper nutrition—can you build vital energy, endurance, and reliable results that last.

The following herbal recommendations are not a quick-loss formula; their purpose is to stabilize a woman's total health while she gains in fitness, assisting willpower, regular physical exertion of some joyful kind, and nature's blueprint for a mature woman's shape. You will find that they reduce food cravings and gas; in addition they increase nutrition during changes in eating and exercising.

Herbal Medicine

GARDEN IN A CUP

Extracts	Botanical Names	Actions
2 oz. rosemary herb	*Rosmarinus officinalis*	Improves circulation; reduces bloating, gas
2 oz. sage leaf	*Salvia officinalis*	Supports hormonal balance; tones bowel wall
1 1/2 oz. wild yam root	*Dioscorea villosa*	Anti-inflammatory; supports hormonal stability
1/2 oz. licorice root	*Glycyrrhiza glabra*	Soothes; stabilizes blood sugar, elimination

Six ounces will last three weeks. Combine these herbal extracts. Take 1/2 teaspoon in 1 cup water, juice, or any herb tea five to thirty minutes before meals.

GARDEN IN A CUP OF TEA

Dried Herbs	Botanical Names	Actions
4 oz. rosemary herb	*Rosmarinus officinalis*	Improves circulation; reduces bloating, gas
4 oz. sage leaf	*Salvia officinalis*	Supports hormonal balance; tones bowel wall
3 oz. wild yam root	*Dioscorea villosa*	Anti-inflammatory; supports hormonal stability
1 oz. licorice root	*Glycyrrhiza glabra*	Soothes; stabilizes blood sugar, elimination

Twelve ounces will last thirty-six days. Add 1/3 ounce of the mixture to 3 cups of boiling water in a teapot or container with a well-fitting lid. Let stand for fifteen minutes before straining. Drink 1 cup hot or cold three times a day five to thirty minutes before meals. Or, if you prefer, sip tea all day or drink two large glasses twice a day, making sure you drink 3 cups in a day.

Nervous System Changes

Lowered estrogen after menopause can make menstrual migraines disappear, but new changes in the nervous system can dim the glorious horizon. It's a little hard to hear about the joy of later years when you haven't slept well because of worry or pain or when you're experiencing some unsettling loss of memory.

Stress seems to increase just when we would welcome a break from the pressure of meeting daily demands. Every woman past middle age has her own set of worries. We worry about our families, our lack of economic security; we care for disabled spouses and parents; we take in our grandchildren when their parents cannot care for them. Because we must take care of ourselves and others, drawing upon all our inner resources, any one of these concerns may bring our own fear of illness out into the open. Fear of losing independence wins all the polls as the most frightening change older women face. For many of us, the loss of an extended family living nearby has added to our sense of isolation. The problem is that these bad feelings can be like a snowball rolling down a hill: they get bigger and bigger, becoming risk factors for depression and lowered immunity.

The changes in our nervous systems do not mean we are losing ourselves. Memory loss, sleep deprivation, and headaches can make anyone feel uncertain of her next move. But this can change. Whatever you have been doing in the past, get in the habits now that you wish to retain into your old age. Actively work at improving positive behaviors with counseling, meditation, or other healing ways.

One important way to cope with stress is to make a list of your problems, put them into order of priority, then list some of the things that can change them and the steps you can take without much effort. They don't have to be big steps, just little ones. Get up tomorrow and do something new or different. Prepare a nourishing meal. Call someone and go on a walk. Volunteer at something you care about. If you are a caregiver, perhaps you can get some occasional help so you can spend some quality time with yourself.

Another thing you can do is to identify the things that turn about over and over in your mind. You may or may not be able to resolve the dilemma, but perhaps you may eventually be able to identify it when it occurs and say to yourself, "There it is again!" Perhaps you may come to accept it or even laugh at it.

Everyone has known someone who aged well and enjoyed what life could offer. Thinking about what you admire and value about that special person may suggest a new path for you to travel, a new adventure to embark upon. Perhaps you have always wanted to do something but never had the time to try it. Now is the time to do it. Women expressing fulfillment during this third of their lives all develop one underlying trait: They are models of an adventurous spirit. Following where your interests lead is the surest path to satisfying your need for physical and mental activity, interacting with interesting ideas or people, and enjoying self-sufficiency.

If nothing seems to work, if you feel as if you are always sad, if you don't want to leave the house, or if you are experiencing memory loss, you need to take care of yourself and get the help you need. Talk to someone: a friend, a family member, a community organization, a trusted health-care practitioner.

Herbal Medicine

Nothing can replace your will to be well, but you can also safely and effectively use natural methods for support in coping with disrupted sleep patterns, loneliness, and a different response to stress. All the formulas in this section contain at least one herbal remedy to help the adrenal glands help you cope with or adapt to stress.

❦——————————— GOOD DAY ———————————❦

Extracts	Botanical Names	Actions
6 oz. ginkgo leaf	*Ginkgo biloba*	Improves memory, mood, blood vessels
4 oz. Siberian gingseng root	*Eleutherococcus senticosus*	Strengthens stress response, immune resistance
2 oz. skullcap herb	*Scutellaria laterifolia*	Relaxes tension; mildly calming

The best results come from consistent use for a minimum of two to three months; good results occur from even short-term use (two to four weeks). A lower dose taken longer is more effective than a high dose taken short term. Twelve ounces will last approximately through the first four weeks.

Combine these herbal extracts. Take 1/4 teaspoon in 1 cup water, juice, or any herb tea three times a day with meals (before or after). This is a mild dose amounting to less than 1 ounce of the formula per week. If you do not notice a change after a week, increase to 1/2 teaspoon in 1 cup of water three times a day with meals. If needed, increase each dose to 1 teaspoon; if you are in good health, you can take a maximum of 2 teaspoons, which is equal to 1 ounce of the formula per day (divided over the day into three doses). If you prefer, put the 2 teaspoons in a full cup of hot water or tea, allow to cool for five or ten minutes, and then drink. This method allows much of the alcohol contained in the extracts to evaporate without destroying the beneficial properties of the herbs. The less alcohol the better, though it is safe to say, after this hot water precaution, the effects of the remaining alcohol are by far outweighed by the benefits of the herbs. Check with your care provider if you have questions.

"Good Day" can be taken for six months; then you should reduce the dose to 1/4 teaspoon or drop the remedy altogether. You'll find that the remedy's benefits last for some time after you stop taking it.

Dried Herbs	Botanical Names	Actions
6 oz. ginkgo leaf	*Ginkgo biloba*	Improves memory, mood, blood vessels
4 oz. Siberian gingseng root	*Eleutherococcus senticosus*	Strengthens stress response, immune resistance
3 oz. lemon balm leaf	*Melissa officinalis*	For taste, digestion; lifts mood
1–2 oz. skullcap herb	*Scutellaria laterifolia*	Relaxes tension; mildly calming
Optional, to taste:		
1/4 oz. ginger	*Zingiber officinale*	Stimulates circulation to brain

See the previous recipe for information about the mixture's benefits and length of use. Again, the most lasting benefits come after several weeks.

Fifteen ounces will last thirty days. Add 1/2 ounce of the mixture to 3 cups of boiling water in a teapot or container with a well-fitting lid. Let stand for fifteen minutes before straining. Drink 1 cup hot or cold twice a day. Because these herbs are lightweight and "fluffy," you may find them easier to handle if you make a big batch once every three days and refrigerate it. Preparing the tea in quantity also allows you to drink more than two cups a day, which is perfectly fine: it's safe, and your body will tell you if you want more on some days. For three days of strong tea, pour 2 quarts of boiling water over 2 ounces of herbs; let the mixture sit, covered, for twenty minutes; then strain and drink as desired. You should enjoy the taste of this tea, so make it as strong or weak as you wish.

When you can't get a good night's sleep, you won't have a good day. Occasional use of herbs can provide temporary relief from sleeplessness or pain and avoid dependence on stronger drugs. The following formulas avoid the possibility of drug interaction, and, taken as directed, are non-habit-forming.

Note that the formulas use valerian, which is not the herbal source for the prescription drug Valium. Biochemically speaking, they have nothing to do with each other. However, if you are being treated for depression or are sensitive to alcohol, ask your health-care provider if you may use the milder tea. Three hints about using valerian: First, it is the best herb for bringing on sleepiness, but some people have the opposite reaction—the sedative alkaloids in the plant make them feel as if they drank too much coffee. If this happens, even once, leave out the valerian. Second, other drugs, prescription or recreational, have the potential to sensitize the nervous system, making it react unpredictably to even small amounts of sedative herbs such as valerian. This reaction can happen to anyone but more frequently to women who have smoked a lot of marijuana. Third, some women find that valerian works well, but if they overdo it, it can leave a dull, hungover feeling upon waking. This can happen from herbal tablets or teas, even those not using extracts containing alcohol. Combining valerian with other herbs to soften its intensity or using alternatives suggested in the formulas allows you to enjoy healing sleep without paying a big price for it the following day.

Some women get great results from the first night onward. Others, especially when they are highly stressed at the start, see improvement after three or four days. "Good Night" also helps with headaches.

❦ ———————————— GOOD NIGHT ———————————— ❦

Extracts	Botanical Names	Actions
4 oz. passion flower herb	*Passiflora incarnata*	Safely inhibits pain; lowers anxiety; helps you stay asleep
2 oz. skullcap herb	*Scutellaria laterifolia*	Relaxes muscle tension; calming
2 oz. valerian root	*Valeriana officinalis*	Helps you get to sleep

Eight ounces will last one to two weeks depending on need. For a change, don't combine these herbal extracts; try a small amount once or twice to see if it works for you. Mix 1/2 teaspoon of passion flower plus 1/4 teaspoon each of skullcap and valerian in 1/3 cup water or juice (white grape juice helps with the peculiar smell and taste). Drink the mixture about twenty minutes before bedtime; repeat dose if needed just before bed and a third time if you awaken sleepless or in pain during the night.

If you find you have a jittery reaction to valerian, leave it out. Combine the herb extracts that agree with you, and take 1 teaspoon of the combination in 1/3 cup liquid as needed.

For temporary pain relief during the day, use smaller amounts: up to 1/2 teaspoon every hour or two as needed. Undiagnosed pain or untreated insomnia that lasts longer than one to two weeks is your signal to check with a care provider.

❦ ———————————— GOOD NIGHT TEA ———————————— ❦

Dried Herbs	Botanical Names	Actions
6 oz. passion flower herb	*Passiflora incarnata*	Safely inhibits pain; lowers anxiety; helps you stay asleep
3 oz. skullcap herb	*Scutellaria laterifolia*	Relaxes muscle tension; calming
3 oz. valerian root	*Valeriana officinalis*	Helps you get to sleep

Twelve ounces will last one to two weeks depending on need. Start by adding 1 ounce of the mixture to 2 1/2 cups of boiling water in a teapot or container with a well-fitting lid. Let stand for fifteen minutes before straining. Drink 1 cup hot or cold an hour before bed; then drink a half cup half an hour before bed, and, if needed, another half cup at bedtime. Remember to empty the bladder last thing before going to bed. You can sip another cup if pain or agitation awaken you during the night. During the day, drink a half cup as needed for temporary pain relief. Any undiagnosed pain or untreated insomnia that lasts longer than one to two weeks is a signal for you to check with a care provider. Valerian may be omitted if you can't get past the taste or if you have any negative sensitivity to it.

Nutrition

Wise Food Choices

- Eat a walnut every day, plain or broken and unheated, in vegetable or grain dishes. Walnuts and many other nuts provide a small amount of essential fatty acids, vegetable protein, vitamins B and E, calcium, iron, potassium, magnesium, and other nutrients. According to folklore, walnuts are associated with better brain power; one a day isn't enough to be fattening.
- Avoid eating dairy foods in excess. Cheese and butter, for example, are loaded with fat and salt, which clog arteries, affecting blood supply everywhere, including the brain.
- If you do not get indigestion from garlic, eat a raw or steamed clove every day to lower cholesterol, help general immunity, and improve circulation, necessary for getting oxygen to the brain.

Supplements

- To add to memory and mental clarity, take gotu kola *(Centella asiatica)*, a bitter-tasting tropical trailing vine available in tablets and as a liquid extract. Use as directed on labels.

In Addition

- Carry a small vial of essential oil of peppermint (available at any drugstore). Place a drop on a cotton ball and place it in the car or near your desk. In aromatherapy experiments, peppermint in factory air vents significantly increased alertness and improved mood.
- Grow a rosemary plant indoors or out. Eat one leaf each day, making sure you chew it slowly. Rub the fragrant leaves between your fingers while on the phone or reading something important. The next time you rub rosemary leaves or sniff its essential oil, your recall will be better.
- Exercise of any type that suits you improves every aspect of mental clarity. Even a slow, stately walk clears the mind, massages the heart, and draws forth hidden wellsprings of inspiration.

Immune Strength

Immunity does not automatically worsen because of age, but it may seem that way, especially if you are exposed daily to children or the public and constantly get colds, flu, and other infections. The following formulas help rebuild your immunity to avoid colds, flus, common urinary-tract infections, and shingles.

Colds and Flus

As you age, you will have a special need to keep minor colds and flus from settling into your lungs to avoid the need for antibiotics or medical care for more serious problems. This is especially true if arthritis limits your chest and upper back muscles from expanding easily. You can alleviate minor conditions on your own; serious infections such as pneumonia require professional care. Most women can distinguish between a common problem and an uncommon medical need, but when common sense causes you to feel doubt, check with a professional.

"Essential Defense," taken either as a combination of extracts or as a tea, can help prevent early signs of illness, especially to keep sore throats and colds from settling in the chest, or can help fight off an already-established infection. It provides a whole-body immune tune-up that covers sinus, lung, throat, stomach, intestinal, and lymph node infections that are not life threatening. "Essential Defense" can be taken along with or after antibiotics, without negative interaction. People may think of echinacea first for any infection, but it isn't necessary to use it every time, and it isn't the best at fighting colds or flus, which is why it is at the bottom of the list for this type of immune system therapy. Include echinacea in the combination only when infections are stubborn or repeated more than twice in a winter.

Herbal Medicine

------------------------- ESSENTIAL DEFENSE -------------------------

Extracts	Botancial Names	Actions
3 oz. sage leaf	*Salvia officinalis*	Relieves sore throats; antiseptic, cleansing
1 oz. yarrow herb	*Achillea millefolium*	Anti-inflammatory; lymph tonic
1 oz. rosemary herb	*Rosmarinus officinalis*	Antiseptic for sinus, lungs, stomach
1 oz. black cohosh root	*Cimicifuga racemosa*	For muscle stiffness, congested lungs

Any or all of the following may be used optionally; vary amounts to taste:

1/4 oz. licorice root	*Glycyrrhiza glabra*	Antiviral; soothing for dry coughs
1/4 oz. ginger root	*Zingiber officinale*	Warming for a cold; settles the stomach
1 oz. echinacea root	*Echinacea* species	Broad-spectrum antimicrobial; immune aid for more stubborn infections

Six to seven ounces will last two to three weeks. Combine these herbal extracts. Take 1 teaspoon in 1 cup water, juice, or any herb tea every hour for the first day or two; then continue, even if feeling better, four times a day, tapering off to twice a day, morning and evening, until two to three weeks are up.

❦ —————— ESSENTIAL DEFENSE TEA —————— ❦

Dried Herbs	Botancial Names	Actions
3 oz. sage leaf	*Salvia officinalis*	Relieves sore throats; antiseptic, cleansing
1 oz. yarrow herb	*Achillea millefolium*	Anti-inflammatory; lymph tonic
2 oz. rosemary herb	*Rosmarinus officinalis*	Antiseptic for sinus, lungs, stomach

Any or all of the following may be used optionally; vary amounts to taste:

1/2 oz. licorice root	*Glycyrrhiza glabra*	Antiviral; soothing for dry coughs
1/4 oz. ginger root	*Zingiber officinale*	Warming for a cold; settles the stomach
1–3 oz. echinacea root	*Echinacea* species	Broad-spectrum antimicrobial; immune aid

Six to ten ounces will last two to three weeks. Add 1 ounce of the mixture to 4 cups boiling water in a teapot or container with a well-fitting lid. Let stand for fifteen minutes before straining. Drink 1/2 cup hot tea every hour for the first day or two (you may reheat a cup at a time at low temperature). Or, if you prefer, sip tea all day, making sure you drink the amount you strained out from the 4 cups of water. Even if you are feeling better, continue to drink 1 cup four times a day for another few days, tapering off to a cup twice a day, morning and evening.

Nutrition

Wise Food Choices

- Eat a clove of raw or lightly steamed or cooked garlic each day for one to two weeks.
- Add a pinch of thyme to broth, soups, or cooked grains daily for three days.
- Add 1 ounce dried or 3 ounces fresh shiitake mushrooms every other day to cooked foods, stir-fried vegetable dishes, soups, broths, and casseroles. These delicious mushrooms are available dried or fresh in Asian produce sections of grocery stores; like many specialized or wild mushrooms, they build non-specific immunity.
- Add a pinch of cayenne (red pepper) to foods for vitamin C and antimicrobial volatile oils to protect against colds. Some hearty older women sprinkle it on salads or brown rice; others stir 1/4 teaspoon in a glass of water at room temperature and knock it back as a daily winter preventative. If cayenne disagrees with your constitution, as with any food or herb, don't force yourself to use it.
- Turmeric, the yellow herb in curry powder blends, is an antioxidant and immune booster. Enjoy frequent curry dishes, adding it according to taste.

Supplements

- Vitamin C with bioflavonoids from food sources (for example, acerola), 2 to 6 grams per day for ten days. Excess vitamin C may cause looseness of stool; if this occurs, reduce or drop dose to bowel tolerance.
- Flax seed oil in capsules or liquid, 1/2 teaspoon per day in easily digested blender drink of your choice (but avoid dairy foods while fighting a cold).
- Grapefruit seed extract taken as directed on labels; or, if citrus agrees with you, eat pieces of the fruit, including a little of the white pithy lining of the rind, for fiber, vitamin C, bioflavonoids, and immune benefits.

In Addition

- A cold is just that—a drop in your temperature. A normal body temperature kills off unwanted germs. When these common microbes are numerous, a raised body temperature is nature's way of cooking the germs. Instead of getting a fever, soak your body in a comfortably hot bath for at least twenty minutes. In the process, you will also be sweating out impurities, lessening the burden on your immune system. Optionally, you may add 5 to 10 drops of one or more of your favorite disinfecting and mood-sweetening essential oils: rose (expensive but a few drops are a powerful and safe disinfectant for all skin types), sandalwood, cedarwood, anise seed, birch, sage, rosemary. Use only 2 to 4 drops of the following stronger oils: lemon, eucalyptus, ti tree, also known as tea tree *(Melaleuca alternifolia, M. quinquenervia).*

- If you don't have a bathtub or if you prefer showers, add these essential oils to shower gels or place drops in the corners of the shower stall for a volatile, cleansing, steamy shower.

- Try this visualization: Drink a cup of herb tea; then sit back in your hot bath or in bed. Imagine ("image in") your white blood cells receiving magic droplets of botanical biochemicals, equipping them to rove out into every place in your body that is tender or hot. See the outsiders—viruses, fungi, and bacteria—stopping in their tracks as your immune cells explain that they must move elsewhere. Subdued and repenting any harm they may have caused, the microbes let their weakened forces be swept into lymph nodes for neutralizing and from there to pathways of excretion for a speedy exit. Recycled as pieces of harmless matter, they are restored to the vast pool of a living Earth to find their rightful spot.

Urinary-Tract Infections

When prescriptions and creams don't work, the following herb formulas can help your own defenses combat cystitis and other common urinary-tract infections. Cystitis is an inflammation of the bladder that usually but not always occurs with an infection. But there is an exception: interstitial cystitis (IC) feels like a urinary-tract infection, but there are no bacteria in the urine. Some doctors believe that in some cases of IC infections actually do occur, but with organisms like chlamydia, which are not usually looked for when cystitis symptoms appear. On the other hand, antibiotics have been considered as one possible cause of IC, as has an allergic type of response. The pain of IC is worse as the bladder fills, so frequent trips to the bathroom are perhaps annoying but advisable. The long-term nature of the problem may not respond quickly to the following herbs, but the formulas below will at least help flush an increased fluid volume through the urinary tract to prevent secondary infections, spasm, and pain. For IC, add to either the extract or tea of "Clear Streams" 1 ounce of nettle leaf *(Urtica dioica),* 1 ounce echinacea root (any *Echinacea* species), and 2 ounces of St. John's wort herb *(Hypericum perforatum).*

The following formulas are designed with the older woman in mind, so they are different from the formulas for cystitis included in Chapter 2, "Menopause." Note that a bladder infection (cystitis) and stress incontinence (weak bladder tone) are not the same, but the following herbal approach will help in either case.

Herbal Medicine

CLEAR STREAMS

Extracts	Botanical Names	Actions
2 oz. marshmallow root	*Althaea officinalis*	Coats and protects vulnerable tissue linings; soothing diuretic
1 oz. passion flower	*Passiflora incarnata*	Reduces pain sensations
2 oz. cramp bark	*Viburnum opulus*	Relaxes spasms; allows urinary stream to follow
2 oz. bearberry leaf	*Arctostaphylos uva-ursi*	Disinfects; stimulates urine flow
1 oz. fresh shepherd's purse	*Capsella bursa-pastoris*	Supports immunity, healing

Eight ounces will last about one week. Combine these herbal extracts. Take 1 teaspoon up to 1 tablespoon in 1 cup water, juice, or any herb tea every hour for one day. Follow with 1 teaspoon in water twice a day until symptoms subside. If any infection does not respond in one week, see your health-care provider. If microbes are still present, continue using the remedy for another two weeks, with monitoring by your health-care provider. These herbs work with or without antibiotics.

CLEAR STREAMS TEA

Dried Herbs	Botanical Names	Actions
3 oz. marshmallow root	*Althaea officinalis*	Coats and protects vulnerable tissue linings; soothing diuretic
3 oz. bearberry leaf	*Arctostaphylos uva-ursi*	Disinfects, stimulates urine flow
1 oz. passion flower	*Passiflora incarnata*	Reduces pain sensations
1 oz. cramp bark	*Viburnum opulus*	Relaxes spasms; allows urinary stream to follow

Eight ounces will last about two weeks. Add 1/2 ounce to 3 1/2 cups of boiling water in a teapot or container with a well-fitting lid. Let stand for fifteen minutes before straining. Drink 1 cup hot or cold three times a day until symptoms subside. If the infection does not respond in one week, see your health-care provider. Continue drinking the tea another week even if antibiotics are needed.

Shingles

Shingles is a completely different infection that becomes more aggravating the older you get. Shingles is caused by a member of the herpes family of viruses that stays dormant in the nerve cells. This is varicella, the same virus that causes chicken pox. It flares up during periods of depressed immunity, including depression and emotional strain. Chronic shingles especially flares up after medical procedures or other stressful experiences. When the virus damages a nerve supplying the skin with sensation, the sensation on the skin is searing pain, and the skin may remain normal or break out in raised red bumps. If scratched, the rash may itch, bleed, or get infected, and it may be too painful to be covered with clothing or a bedsheet. When it is possible to use remedies on the surface, such as at the very first warning sign, tingling pain, you can apply external remedies to the skin (see "In Addition").

Although no herb is known to get rid of shingles or other herpes infections entirely, the following formula contains antiviral herbs that restore strength and immune resistance to the nerve tissues. You can take it for a few weeks or even a few months at a time for prevention as well as treatment during outbreaks.

If you have high blood pressure or a weak heart or kidneys, replace licorice root with an equal amount of suma *(Pfaffia paniculata)* or Siberian ginseng *(Eleutherococcus senticosus)*. Suma is an expensive immunity-building herb from the Amazonian rain forest but worth the cost if you can get the root in the form of an extract or tea. It is not endangered. Siberian ginseng has immunity-building and stress-reducing properties and does not have the overstimulating side effects sometimes seen with ginseng.

❦ ——————————————— SHINGLE-FREE COMPOUND ——————————————— ❦

Extracts	Botanical Names	Actions
4 oz. St. John's wort herb	*Hypericum perforatum*	Antiviral; repairs nerves; antidepressant
4 oz. licorice root	*Glycyrrhiza glabra*	Antiviral; anti-inflammatory; harmonizes
2 oz. passion flower herb	*Passiflora incarnata*	Decreases pain sensitivity; relaxes

Ten ounces will last about fifteen days. Combine these herbal extracts. Take 2 teaspoons in 1 cup water, juice, or any herb tea each morning and evening. Extra doses of 1 teaspoon may be taken to relieve symptoms between regular doses.

Dried Herbs	Botanical Names	Actions
4 oz. St. John's wort herb	*Hypericum perforatum*	Antiviral; repairs nerves; anti-depressant
2 oz. echinacea root	*Echinacea* species	Antimicrobial; helps lymph, immunity
2 oz. passion flower herb	*Passiflora incarnata*	Decreases pain sensitivity; relaxes
1 oz. skullcap herb	*Scutellaria laterifolia*	Unwinds emotional tension
1 oz. licorice root	*Glycyrrhiza glabra*	Antiviral; anti-inflammatory; harmonizes

Ten ounces will last from fifteen to twenty-one days. Add 1 ounce of the mixture to 4 cups of boiling water in a teapot or container with a well-fitting lid. Let stand for twenty minutes before straining. Drink 1 cup warm or cool four times a day for two days. Then add 1/2 ounce to 3 cups boiling water; let sit twenty minutes or until room temperature. Drink 1 cup twice a day for the next week. Extra doses of a half cup may be taken to ease symptoms between regular doses.

Nutrition

Wise Food Choices

- Eat 4 to 7 ounces grilled or broiled flounder or other white fish one to two times a week or during periods of higher stress.
- Eat 1 to 3 cloves raw garlic a day, or as many as you can tolerate at the first tingling sensation or during outbreaks.
- Avoid peanuts, chocolate, and coffee, which are rich in chemicals that promote herpes flare-ups.

Supplements

- 500 milligrams of lysine, an amino acid, to help prevent outbreaks of the shingles virus
- Garlic tablets or perles, plain or deodorized, if dietary form unappealing (250 to 750 milligrams daily)

In Addition

- Apply the following external herb oil for temporary pain numbing and anti-viral and anti-itch properties. Combine in a plastic cosmetic bottle with a spray top: 1 ounce St. John's wort oil (available at herb shops or from the mail-order outlets listed in "Resources") and 1/4 ounce essential oil of peppermint (available at many drugstores); for added strength, you can add pressed juice of two garlic cloves. Store in the refrigerator for up to six months.

If the oils break down the plastic, store in glass until needed or switch to new container. (If you can find them, glass bottles with sprayers are preferable.) Spray a light mist on painful skin as needed. It doesn't need to be rubbed in, but it will stain clothing and smell strongly of mint (and garlic if added).

Skin Changes

There is every reason you can maintain or reattain lovely, healthy skin after menopause. The change in tone at this age is due to loss of elasticity and water within the cell. Expensive products rubbed in externally may go only so far. Natural substances may not turn back the hands of time, but they will soften your hands and face, smooth the worst of your wrinkles back to fine lines, and tone circulation, which in turn brings improved tone to skin, fat layers, muscle tissue, and your movement through space.

Note: Women beyond menopause often worry that any little skin change may mean cancer. Considering all the risk factors we face with age, our concern is not unreasonable. Signs and symptoms are your body's way of telling you to pay attention now rather than ignoring a change in the hope it will go away, and then ignoring it because you fear what it may mean. It is wise to seek a qualified opinion if a new spot appears on your face, neck, or hands, or if a mole or bump changes size or color or becomes sore.

The following remedies are known for their gentle, supportive ability to tone the skin from the inside out. They may be taken from time to time for healthy skin maintenance, or they may be used for a short, intensive spell to begin repair and renewal in the case of varicose veins, age spots, thin skin, and other cosmetic challenges. The recommended herbs are only one aspect of the best holistic self-care. Consult with an experienced massage therapist, aromatherapist (skilled in the use of essential oils), or other person qualified to do facials (ideally one skilled in acupressure for natural facelifts and techniques that help problem areas such as bags under the eyes or deep lines).

Herbal Medicine

❧ ——————————————— AGELESS BEAUTY ——————————————— ❧

Extracts	Botanical Names	Actions
4 oz. sarsaparilla root	*Smilax ornata*	Tones skin, lymph; supports immunity
2 oz. dong quai root	*Angelica sinensis*	Builds healthy blood; warming
1 oz. nettle leaf	*Urtica dioica*	Mineralizing; nutritive
1/2 oz. horsetail herb	*Equisetum arvense*	Tones kidneys, skin
1/4 oz. yellow dock root	*Rumex crispus*	Cleanses liver; clears skin
1/4 oz. calendula flower	*Calendula officinalis*	Liver, lymph, skin tonic

Eight ounces will last just over three weeks. Combine these herbal extracts. Take 1 teaspoon in 1 cup water, juice, or any herb tea three times a day. Take for at least three days at a time for maintenance, up to three weeks or so. For long-term tonic benefits, use one of the following easy methods: Take three times a day five days out of each week, skipping weekends, as long as your skin keeps improving (three to twelve months); or take only twice a day up to three months before taking a break of two to four weeks, repeating the regimen as long as your skin keeps improving and the herbs agree with your system.

AGELESS BEAUTY BEVERAGE

Dried Herbs	Botanical Names	Actions
6 oz. sarsaparilla root	*Smilax ornata*	Tones skin, lymph; supports immunity
3 oz. dong quai root	*Angelica sinensis*	Builds healthy blood; warming
2 oz. nettle leaf	*Urtica dioica*	Mineralizing; nutritive
1 oz. horsetail herb	*Equisetum arvense*	Tones kidneys, skin
1/2 oz. yellow dock root	*Rumex crispus*	Cleanses liver; clears skin
1/2 oz. calendula flower	*Calendula officinalis*	Liver, lymph, skin tonic

Fourteen ounces will last about three weeks. Add 3/4 ounce of the mixture to 4 cups of boiling water in a teapot or container with a well-fitting lid. Let stand for twenty minutes before straining. Drink 1 cup hot or cold four times a day. Or, if you prefer, drink two large glasses twice a day, making sure as you drink 4 cups a day. The extra water is as important as the herbs for healthy skin.

Nutrition

Wise Food Choices

- Eat one large carrot or drink 4 to 8 ounces fresh carrot juice at least three times a week.
- Eat dark green vegetables.
- Eat at least two pieces of whole, fresh, organic fruit in season per day.

Supplements

- Vitamin E, 200 to 800 I.U. per day
- Vitamin A or beta-carotene according to product labels, staying within a conservative daily dose
- Evening primrose oil and other GLA (gamma linoleic acid) supplements (borage seed oil, black currant seed oil) as directed on labels or up to 12 capsules a day: 4 capsules taken with food three times a day

In Addition

- Go without anything on your skin (even natural products) for a whole day and night to see how it feels. Even pure herbal moisturizers have reactions. Give your pores a complete "fast" before starting something new.
- Dab a drop of rosewood essential oil on blemishes overnight or under foundation by day.
- The world's simplest bath oil: Add to your bath a capful (about two teaspoons) of just *one* of the following: grape seed oil, avocado oil, walnut oil, sesame oil. Do not add a scent. Allow the silky water to coat every inch of you; rub it into dry places. Avoid using soap, at least just for this bath. Wash hair in the water; don't rinse; leave on overnight as a hot-oil treatment for your scalp; shampoo in shower next morning. When getting out of bath, simply pat dry; don't rub. Be careful not to slip when stepping out of tub.
- External massage blend for wrinkles: Mix 1/4 ounce vitamin E oil with 1 ounce almond, sesame, walnut, or avocado oil. *Optional:* Add one or more essential oils according to personal preference: 2 drops neroli (orange blossom), 2 drops geranium, 1 drop sandalwood. Making gentle, circular motions with fingertips, massage oil in skin or face, skin, and hands. This blend is especially good for moisturizing after washing or bathing or before bed.
- Rediscover astringent and nondrying witch hazel (available at any drugstore). Pat face and neck, especially broken capillaries, after baths, showers, exercise, and saunas. For varicose veins, wrap towels soaked in refrigerator-cold witch hazel around legs. Rest with legs elevated slightly at least twenty minutes a day or as needed.
- Make an herbal skin toner without alcohol: Steep 1 ounce dried nettle in 2 cups just-boiled water for twenty minutes. Strain; while nettle tea is still warm but not hot, add 15 drops essential oil of blue chamomile or 5 drops each of neroli, rosewood, frankincense, and palmarosa essential oils, all of which are highly beneficial to mature and sensitive skin. If one or two are unavailable in your area, use what is available, or substitute one (only one) of the following (depending on the scent you prefer): clary sage, sandalwood, vetiver (from the roots of fragrant grasses). Store in a sterilized plastic bottle near sink (not glass, to avoid breakage); apply with unbleached cotton or clean fingertips (not facial or toilet tissues made from wood pulp—they irritate skin). Rinse with plain, cool water; pat dry. Repeat every day for three days, then once a week as needed.
- Dry skin brushing helps all skin types. You can slough off dry, dead skin cells with a rough wash cloth or a loofah (a natural sponge), which also invigorates blood supply to the skin and releases superficial tension in the muscles. Avoid scrubbing too hard; skin should tingle pleasantly, not burn.

- Exercise. Working up a sweat triggers glandular function and removes impurities. Always choose exercises that you enjoy and that are appropriate to your current state of health.
- Apply an external facial blend (see box).

External Facial Blend

For difficult-to-treat, blotchy skin with dry, oily, reddened areas and broken capillaries, mix together:

1 oz. sesame oil
10 drops essential oil of cypress
5 drops essential oil of thyme
5 drops essential oil of marjoram
5 drops essential oil of geranium

Store mixed oils in a glass bottle with a lid that is easy to tighten and remove each day. Dropper tops are fine, but oils break down the rubber seal after a while. To use: Wash face and neck with plain warm water; dry lightly. Place a liberal amount (about a teaspoon) in one hand; use fingers of other hand to spread oils in circular motions on skin. Avoid getting too close to eyes and mouth: it doesn't taste good on lips but won't hurt you. Massage in generously (but without pulling at skin) for a full five minutes. It takes this long to penetrate several layers of skin, stimulate self-cleansing, and relax tight facial muscles. To rinse, splash repeatedly with plain, cold water, which will remove excess oil, tone tiny blood vessels, and tighten pores. Pat dry with a soft towel. Repeat every day for a minimum of twenty days and see the difference! Repeat once every week or two as needed.

Vaginal Changes

More than ever before, postmenopausal women are beginning new relationships, so a new love in your sixties or later shouldn't surprise anyone. There's no mystery to having good sex during this stage of life. In health, humans can enjoy sex as long as they keep the pump primed. When age-related problems get in the way of your enjoyment, acceptance of the situation, taking your time, and using herbal remedies can make all the difference.

Among postmenopausal women, two primary obstacles to good sex are vaginal dryness and atrophy. If you feel pain while having sex, vaginal dryness is the probable cause (see Chapter 2). It may occur because the contents of the pelvis have dropped, especially if there is a loss of tone. Postmenopausal thinning, or atrophy, may take up to ten years to show up and is different from vaginal dryness. After menopause, the labia minora (Latin for "little lips," the folds of skin enclosing the vaginal opening) may disappear, while the labia majora (the larger, outer pair of vaginal lips) become thinner. The vagina itself becomes smaller, the linings thinner and less "tough." As a result, irritations and infections may become chronic and immune defense less abundant, especially if circulation and nutrition are poor.

The supportive ligaments of the pelvis lose some of their tone, becoming more vulnerable to prolapse (dropping down out of place). Moreover, starting at the onset of menopause, the cervix slowly decreases in size, and the secretory glands it contains may become less active with less sexual stimulation. Because the uterine lining stops thickening and shedding in a monthly cycle, and the uterus knows it won't have to push another infant into the world now, the muscle layer of the uterus thins. But not to worry: This change is not problematic as long as you take care to maintain health and guard against minor infections, abrasions, inflammations, and dry spells—conditions that our vaginas could ignore fifteen years ago and now more likely to get our full attention.

Maintaining natural lubrication protects you from infections caused by microbes, even sneaky ones that can exploit a lack of immunity at this doorway to the body, rising up the urethral opening in the vagina and possibly leading to bladder infections (see the section on urinary-tract infections in "Immune Strength," earlier in this chapter). Because these vaginal infections involve both the reproductive and urinary tracts, the natural methods for preventing or treating them utilize herbs with an affinity for both body systems. It is a revelation to study the qualities of such doubly helpful herbs, only to realize that some of them are hormonal normalizing tonics as well. Nature has certainly provided for us!

The use of "Nourishing Paradise" tea over three to six months improves vaginal tissue health by preventing infections caused by dryness even though vaginal walls may be thinner. The herbs cannot guarantee a lack of infection but can add gentle anti-inflammatory and healing properties to the skin's natural immune defenses. The tea can be used in addition to, or after short-term use of, the extract elixir below.

Herbal Medicine

GOLDEN PANTHER POTION

Extracts	Botanical Names	Actions
4 oz. red clover flower	*Trifolium pratense*	Nutritive; diuretic; provides minerals, phytoestrogens
2 oz. yarrow flower	*Achillea millefolium*	Astringent; antimicrobial diuretic tonic
1 oz. damiana herb	*Turnera diffusa*	Nervine tonic for energy and genitalia
1 oz. dong quai root	*Angelica sinensis*	Optimizes estrogen, immunity
2 oz. ginseng root	*Panax* species	Increases endurance; lessens fatigue; supports long-term immunity and sexual vitality

Ten ounces will last two weeks to thirty days. Combine these herbal extracts. Take 1 teaspoon in 1 cup water, juice, or any herb tea three times a day for at least two weeks. Best results are seen in three to four weeks. *Note:* If you experience any spotting postmenopausally or note blood in the urine, consult your health-care provider; meanwhile, add 2 ounces fresh plant extract of shepherd's purse *(Capsella bursa-pastoris)* and 2 ounces echinacea extract *(Echinacea* species) to the mixture, increasing the dose to 2 teaspoons four times a day for a minimum of three days even if spotting improves. Don't neglect a medical diagnosis even if herbs seem to clear this symptom.

NOURISHING PARADISE

Dried Herbs	Botanical Names	Actions
3 oz. raspberry leaf	*Rubus idaeus*	Hormone tonic; astringent; diuretic
3 oz. fennel seeds	*Foeniculum vulgare*	Provides phytoestrogens; for taste
2 oz. damiana herb	*Turnera diffusa*	Nervine tonic for energy and genitalia
2 oz. peppermint leaf	*Mentha piperita*	For taste, digestion of above herbs
Optional:		
1 oz. bearberry leaf	*Arctostaphylos uva-ursi*	Astringent; diuretic tonic
1 oz. licorice root	*Glycyrrhiza glabra*	Lubricating; balances moisture of tissue surfaces

Ten ounces will last thirty days. Add 1/3 ounce of the mixture to 3 cups of boiling water in a teapot or container with a well-fitting lid. Let stand for ten to fifteen minutes before straining. Drink 1 cup hot or cold two to three times a day for at least two weeks, at most one month, and then take a break for a few days. Repeat as often or as long as you like. Can be enjoyed by either gender. If taken longer than three months, skip one or two days per week.

Nutrition

Wise Food Choices
- Eat soybeans and soy foods for increased lubrication and fiber. Cook whole soybeans with fennel, celery seeds, cilantro, and other aromatic culinary herbs to improve their digestibility.
- Please also see the recommendations under "Vaginal Thinning and Dryness" in Chapter 2, "Menopause." You can use the same nutritional recommendations and external remedies for postmenopausal dryness and thinning.

MATERIA MEDICA

ALFALFA. *Medicago sativa.* **Part used:** Herb.

Indications: Alfalfa is used to optimize estrogen levels especially when there is also a need to increase vitamins and protein and alter chronic health conditions. It is given long term for arthritis management and helps reduce water retention without stressing the kidneys.

Tea: 2 ounces per pint or quart, infused, taken three times a day (5 to 10 grams per dose).

Tincture: 1 to 2 teaspoons (5 to 10 milliliters) diluted in water, three times a day.

AMERICAN GINSENG. *Panax quinquefolius.* **Part used:** Root. This rare beauty of the Araliaceae family is a different medicinal herb than Chinese or Asian ginseng (*P. ginseng*) though it is used similarly and contains similar constituents in varying concentrations depending on growth, harvesting time, and preparation; see GINSENG, below.

Before the 1960s and 1970s, when the medicinal value of ginseng became known in the West, botanical traders in Asia purchased huge shipments of American ginseng. In the 1960s, when Americans regained interest in herbs and ginseng in particular, Asian ginseng was usually imported to the United States and for a while American ginseng was the preferred species used in China. American ginseng is now endangered in the wild, especially in its main stronghold, the Appalachian Mountains, primarily because of strip mining, overdevelopment, and overharvesting to meet market demand for the herb. To be ecologically responsible, purchase cultivated, "woods-grown," stock, not "wildcrafted" stock harvested from the wild.

Indications: American ginseng is less heating than Asian ginseng and is therefore given to bring down fevers and inflammation of the lungs or digestion. In some Native American cultures where ginseng was available, men and women drank infusions of the root to promote fertility, women chewed on the root for easier labor and delivery, and both men and women took it to stimulate mental clarity. Among Native Americans it was also given to the elderly to increase endurance through the eastern winters. It is not as likely as Asian ginseng to cause dizziness in people who take it without really needing it (see GINSENG). It is a stronger digestive tonic than Asian ginseng, though the latter is also effective.

American ginseng is not associated with toxicity, but because of its tonic effects on labor and delivery, it is best to avoid it during pregnancy unless it is used under a midwife's supervision at low to moderate dosages in the third trimester or last two weeks of pregnancy.

Tea: 1/2 to 2 teaspoons (1 to 4 grams) per cup, infused, one to four times a day.

Tincture: Minimum of 10 drops to 1/2 teaspoon, up to 1 to 2 teaspoons (1 to 2 milliliters, up to 5 to 10 milliliters), diluted in water, taken one to three times a day.

APOTHECARY'S ROSE. See ROSE

BEARBERRY, also called UVA-URSI. *Arctostaphylos uva-ursi.* **Part used:** The small, leathery green leaves are harvested in spring and summer.

Indications: Bearberry is a specific remedy for cystitis, urethritis, and pyelitis (kidney infection); but see "Contraindications," below. In Europe, bearberry is also used for arthritis, gout, and rheumatism because it may stimulate excretion of uric acid.

Bearberry works by disinfecting urine being formed in the kidneys, stored in the bladder, or excreted through the urethra. It is especially helpful when the pH of the urine is alkaline, which can be easily measured at home with pH paper from any drugstore. If urine is acidic, switch to a dairy- and meat-free diet during natural treatments, or take bearberry tea with a pinch of bicarbonate of soda (baking soda). For best results, take the last dose about four hours before bedtime and void the bladder before sleeping to avoid nighttime waking. Also, use up tincture in the days following an infection rather than storing it; the herb's constituents begin breaking down over six to eight months, and the herb will continue to tone the urinary tract against recurrence of infection.

Contraindications: Bearberry is contraindicated in chronic pyelonephritis or any kidney inflammation and also during pregnancy as it may be more irritating than can be tolerated in these conditions.

Tea: 2 grams per dose or 1 teaspoon per cup, up to the "strong, stronger, strongest" dose of 1 tablespoon leaves to 1 cup water, 1 ounce per pint or 3 cups; take 1 cup two to three times a day. Cold infusions of the leaf (steeped in cold water for four hours) are best in order to avoid excess tannins in stubborn cases of cystitis or whenever the herb is used longer than one week at a time. It is best taken for less than six weeks so that high tannins do not interfere with absorption of other minerals. After a break of a few weeks, it can be repeated as before.

Tincture: 1/2 teaspoon (2 1/2 milliliters) diluted in 1 cup water, two to three times per day.

BLACK HAW. See CRAMP BARK

BLACK SNAKEROOT. See BLACK COHOSH

BLACK COHOSH, also called BLACK SNAKEROOT. *Cimicifuga racemosa*. **Parts used:** Root and rhizome (the underground stem). The root and rhizome are hard and knotty, their twisted shape giving the plant its other name, "black snake-root." The name "cohosh" is all this herb has in common with blue cohosh. They are not interchangeable herbs but can be used together.

Indications: Black cohosh is used to optimize estrogen levels although its exact mechanism is still debated. Black cohosh may compete with estrogen receptor sites when estrogen is overabundant but may promote estrogen production when estrogen is low. It is a prime women's tonic for any uterine condition involving inflammation, pain, or low estrogen. It promotes fertility and softens the impact of the Change. It lowers blood pressure by opening up peripheral circulation. In tests black cohosh has been shown to be anti-inflammatory, and it lowers high blood sugar. In addition, Native Americans traditionally used it for all lung congestion, arthritic aches and pains, and nervous coughs. Traditional Chinese medicine employs other *Cimicifuga* species for infectious illnesses and tissue deterioration.

Contraindications: Use of black cohosh is contraindicated in pregnancy except when supervised by experienced midwives and herbalists as an antispasmodic to prevent threatened miscarriage or to coordinate muscular contractions or assist labor. In large doses, over 2 teaspoons, black cohosh may cause headaches.

Tea: Up to 1 ounce (1/4 to 1 teaspoon, or 0.5 to 2 grams) per day, decocted.

Tincture: 1/2 to 1 teaspoon (2 to 5 milliliters) three times a day.

BLADDERWRACK. *Fucus vesiculosus*. **Part used:** Whole plant (seaweed harvested from less-polluted coasts).

Indications: Used as a source of iodine, important to thyroid functions; used for stabilizing appetite, improving metabolism; benefits those working to reduce excess weight. Contains mucopolysaccharides, fiber, and minerals.

Note: The smell of the ocean may not appeal to some women, so using capsules or eating seaweeds is an alternative to using it in herbal combinations.

Tea: 1 to 4 teaspoons (2 to 8 grams) per cup, 1/2 to 2 ounces per pint, infused, taken three times a day.

Tincture: 1 teaspoon (5 milliliters) diluted in water or juice, two to four times a day.

BLUE COHOSH. *Caulophyllum thalictroides*. **Part used:** Root.

Indications: Blue cohosh is a paradoxical herb: it can either stimulate a uterus to contract or inhibit contractions. It is used for amenorrhea (lack of menstrual periods) in women whose cycles are blocked by physical congestion or nervous or hormonal imbalance rather than malnutrition or pregnancy. It is not a definite abortifacient—that is, it is a mistake to try to use it that way. It is used in early pregnancy to prevent miscarriages, though for this use it is usually taken in small doses combined with other antispasmodics such as cramp bark *(Viburnum opulus)* or black haw *(V. prunifolium)*. Its other important use is as a hormonal and tissue toner. Blue cohosh is given along with uterine astringent tonics for tears or surgical damage to the reproductive system during, but especially after, chronic reproductive infections; it also helps shrink fibroids or growths and promotes fertility.

Contraindications: Though it has been called "squaw root" and "papoose root," blue cohosh is contraindicated in pregnancy except when its use is supervised by experienced herbalists or midwives in special circumstances: to prevent miscarriage from the third to the ninth month, when it is used for its antispasmodic action; or to promote easy delivery at the end of term, when it helps coordinate uterine contractions. It may overstimulate a healthy uterus in the first trimester. Midwives and herbalists use it with respectful appreciation for its potency in the right situation at the right dose.

Tea: Other than in pregnancy, the adult dose is 1 to 2 teaspoons (2 to 4 grams) per cup, up to 2 ounces per pint decocted, 1 cup three times a day.

Tincture: 1 teaspoon (5 milliliters) in water, three times a day.

BLUE VERVAIN. See VERVAIN

BORAGE. *Borago officinalis.* **Parts used:** Flower; also leaf, stem.

Indications: The whole plant is anti-inflammatory and calming, in part because of the gel-like starches, or mucilage, it contains. Borage is given in cases of adrenal exhaustion or physical and emotional breakdown. According to modern Chinese research, its steroidal saponins may have an affect on adrenal cortical function. Borage is cooling, so it is given in fevers or infections where chronic debility allows poor immune resistance to flare up into illness. It is especially suited for children's raging fevers. Its softening qualities on heavy hearts and hot fevers also benefit congested lungs; the mucilage and saponins are expectorant and clearing in cases of bronchitis. It has been used in pneumonia. Juice of the whole flowering herb is used for depression. Borage also makes a wonderful syrup or fresh plant glycerin extract. The fresh herb is always better and the flowers are more active than the leaf, so a mixture of two-thirds flowers and one-third leaf and cut stem is most desirable. In past times in Europe, it was one of the herbs strewn on floors for happy social events.

Tea: Dried flowering herb, up to 1 to 2 ounces (3 to 6 grams) infused per pint, 1 cup three times a day.

Tincture: 1 teaspoon to 1 tablespoon diluted in water, three times a day.

CALENDULA, also called POT MARIGOLD. *Calendula officinalis.* **Parts used:** Petal or whole flower head of the nonhybridized, single-headed flower, collected and dried carefully in shade during the peak of flowering. Calendula is used internally as a tea or extract made from the fresh or dried flowers. Petals are used like saffron in cooking or tossed raw in salads and soups for their delicate flavor and immune-strengthening effect. Use a light hand; too many at once are bitter tasting.

Indications: Systemic infections, especially affecting the nerves, skin, or lymph nodes. Calendula is used for flus and fevers, and it improves lymphatic circulation. It is used to clear cystic acne, sebaceous cysts, and chronic imbalance of skin conditions of an autoimmune nature, such as psoriasis. It is a warming and drying herb. Calendula contains many plant pigments that, like the beta-carotene in carrots, make it an effective immune helper with antiviral effects. As it is a lymphatic cleansing agent with a broad antimicrobial range, calendula is an excellent choice in any preparation intended to correct chronic infection. It has been found especially effective against gram-positive bacteria, and even *Trichomonas vaginalis*, a finding discovered by gynecologists in the 1950s and 1960s.

Calendula promotes granulation cell formation, which speeds the knitting together of damaged tissues. It is therefore useful internally and externally for burns, lost tissue, badly healing wounds, and ulcers. Fresh juice has been used by the tablespoon internally and on breast or skin cancers in European nature cure clinics. The Dutch combine it with cow parsley (*Heraclium* species) for this use. Tea, tincture, juice, capsules, and compresses are used internally and externally to decrease hard lymph nodes in cancer. Postoperatively, calendula is given to help prevent metastases.

Tea: 2 teaspoons dried petals or 4 grams dried flowers steeped in 1 cup boiling water for ten to twenty minutes, tightly covered to prevent loss of the herb's fragile components and trace volatile oils. Strain and drink 1 to 4 cups a day as needed. The taste is bitter, so an alcohol-water tincture or fresh plant glycerin extract is often more acceptable.

Tincture: 10 drops to 1/3 teaspoon (1 to 2 milliliters), up to 1/2 to 2 teaspoons, diluted in 1 cup water; take one to four times a day. There is no known toxicity, and up to 1 ounce tincture per week can be used indefinitely. A low dose of 15 to 30 drops of tincture is used hourly for gastrointestinal inflammation such as enteritis and ulceration. Diluting the tincture in a cup of infused marshmallow and calendula tea provides demulcent mucilage to offset any irritation from the high alcohol necessary to extract and preserve the herb's more fragile components. For external or vaginal use, pack fresh flowers in almond, olive, or other vegetable oil; place the mixture on a sunny windowsill or in a warm place, keeping it out of direct light, for ten days or until the oil is a deep golden-orange and fragrant; then strain. This oil can be used directly on dry skin or inflamed areas, and it may be incorporated into lotions or salves for external, rectal, or vaginal use. Rubbing the oil into new bruises quickens their healing.

CHAMOMILE, CAMOMILE, GERMAN CHAMOMILE. *Matricaria recutita*, also *M. chamomilla*. **Parts used:** Flower, flowering herb, essential (volatile) oil.

Indications: Though bitter herbs such as chamomile offer cooling effects by bringing increased blood flow from the body's surface to the central digestive organs, chamomile may also be warming because it brings blood flow to inflamed areas, including the reproductive organs, mucous membranes, and skin. It is given for pain, insomnia, dysmenorrhea, menstrual cramps, PMS (premenstrual syndrome), depression, irritability, intestinal parasites, anorexia, and vertigo. Dilute chamomile tea is given to babies for relief of colic and teething discomfort; at regular strength it is used for diarrhea and upset stomach in children. It is used externally in compresses for conjunctivitis, inflamed skin infections, wounds or rashes, boils, itchy skin of various causes, and *pruritus vulvus*, that dreadful itchiness of the vagina that occurs with or without infection. A few drops of the essential oil in a hot bath can ease stress and pain; use 2 drops for babies and small children, up to 10 or more drops for adults. The herb is a common ingredient in hair rinses for blonds and other fair-haired people and as a facial cleanser for all skin types.

Used externally or internally, chamomile stimulates the formation of healthy new tissue over wounds while it disinfects them. Used internally, this same vulnerary effect combines with chamomile's antispasmodic effect to be useful in healing chronic ulceration. Large doses of chamomile can even sedate smooth (involuntary) muscle, and though it is bitter, it uniquely inhibits excess peristalsis of the digestive tract.

Chamomile is specific for chronic inflammation, constipation, intestinal gas pains, spastic colon, pyloric spasm, diverticulitis, colitis, and all conditions worsened by stress and nervousness. It is given after vomiting to settle the stomach, and it is safe in pregnancy for morning sickness. The primary anti-inflammatory constituent is considered to be azulene, which is not present in fresh herb but is formed from precursors by heat and water. Simple tea is one way to catalyze the precursor into the active form.

When making or buying tincture, make sure the water portion of the extraction method is done with hot water and the mixture cooled down before alcohol or glycerin is added for complete preservation.

Contraindications: Someone who is sensitive to ragweeds and chrysanthemums may be allergic to this calming herb. Though the press has made a big deal out of a few recent cases, the German government and the U.S. Food and Drug Administration generally consider chamomile to be safe. The azulenes have even been shown to have an antiallergic effect by reducing histamine release. It has been suggested that related species more likely to cause allergic reactions may have been substituted in commerce for chamomile, so proper identification and purity of herb or herb products can minimize problems. If skin rash or allergic symptoms appear, discontinue use.

Tea: 1 to 2 teaspoons (2 to 4 grams) per cup, up to 2 ounces per 3 cups, infused; take 3 cups a day. This herb does not extract fully in glycerin.

Tincture: As few as 5 drops of properly prepared tincture (see above) are often effective. The dose ranges from 5 drops to 1/2 to 1 teaspoon diluted in water, taken three times a day. Amounts of 1 1/2 ounces tincture per week or more are used for stubborn problems.

CHASTEBERRY. *Vitex agnus-castus.* **Parts used:** Seed or berry, picked when ripe in the autumn and dried in part sun, part shade.

Indications: Through apparently opposite effects, chasteberry normalizes female sex hormones, especially by lowering excess estrogen. It works via the pituitary to support the function of the progesterone-secreting corpus luteum of ovaries. It is used for dysmenorrhea and premenstrual tension, and it is especially beneficial during menopausal changes. Because it promotes a healthy estrogen-to-progesterone balance, it is used to quicken a return to natural rhythms after use of the birth control pill and to decrease fibrocystic breast tissue. In women without ovaries, chasteberry appears to lessen extremes of hormonal imbalance, perhaps through indirect effects on the endocrine system, liver, and circulation. In large doses (2 ounces tincture daily) it works as an anaphrodisiac in men, explaining its older European name, monkspepper. Some women report an increased sex drive after use of chasteberry; others using this herb who experience a decrease in sexual desire may not have a need for this herb.

Combinations: Though it primarily works by increasing progesterone in cases of deficiency, chasteberry has been used with estrogen-promoting herbs such as dong quai *(Angelica sinensis)* and black cohosh *(Cimicifuga racemosa)* to balance both hormones.

Tea: 1 to 2 teaspoons (2 to 4 grams) crushed seeds steeped in 1 cup boiling water, covered, for ten to fifteen minutes. Doses for therapeutic effects range from 1/2 ounce per pint to 1 ounce per 3 cups, take 1 cup three times a day. Taking the first dose early in the morning upon waking, in place of coffee or other caffeine beverages, has been found to be most helpful.

Tincture: 1/2 to 1 teaspoon (2 1/2 to 5 milliliters) diluted in water; take three times a day.

CINNAMON. *Cinnamomum* species. **Part used:** Inner peeled bark (quills).

Indications: Cinnamon bark is used for reducing nausea, upset stomach, and intestinal bloating and gas. It is given to warm people who are sensitive to cold chills, and it reduces high blood pressure, inflammations, and cramps. It has been used for thousands of years as a woman's remedy. Cinnamon is also given to aid digestion and flavor other medicinal preparations.

Tea: 1/2 to 1 teaspoon (1 to 2 grams) per cup, up to 1 ounce per pint, infused, 1/2 cup three times a day.

Tincture: 1/2 teaspoon (1/2 milliliter) diluted in water, three times a day.

CLARY SAGE, also called CLARY. *Salvia sclarea.* **Parts used:** Flower, leaf, essential oil; sometimes seed.

Indications: The flowers and leaves are made into a "sun tea" given by the glassful for depression and sadness. The seeds have a demulcent quality and have been used as a soothing eye preparation applied in a compress with a tea of whole herb.

Tea: 1 to 2 teaspoons (2 to 4 grams) per cup, 1/2 to 1 ounce in a pint, infused; take 1 cup three times a day.

Tincture: 1/2 to 1 teaspoon (2 1/2 to 5 milliliters) diluted in water, three times a day. Breathe in the essential oil, which has aromatherapy value, throughout the day and evening, or massage 2 to 10 drops essential oil into skin daily. For balancing hormones and relieving depression, a total of 10 drops is applied as a daily massage into wrists, armpits, and temples, where thinner skin and nearby blood vessels allow absorption of volatile oils.

CLOVER. See RED CLOVER

COHOSH. See BLACK COHOSH, BLUE COHOSH

CRAMP BARK, also called GUELDER ROSE or HIGHBUSH CRANBERRY. *Viburnum opulus.* **Parts used:** Bark; also berry (cooked).

Indications: Cramp bark is given for pain caused by tense, contracted muscles, such as with muscle spasms. It is particularly given for involuntary muscle tension (in the womb, stomach, lungs) but affects voluntary muscle as well (in the legs, arms, back, shoulders, neck). Black haw *(V. prunifolium),* another species, may be used for its more local antispasmodic effects on the uterus, fallopian tubes, and surrounding muscles.

Cramp bark is a simple muscle relaxer that operates without any narcotic or mental or emotional sedation. This makes it useful for menstrual cramps or other muscle spasms. It can be given for sports injuries and the clenched-teeth body rigidity of intense pain. Because it relaxes muscles anywhere in high enough doses, it is given to reduce high blood pressure or allergic and asthmatic tightness of the chest. The whole-herb preparations are not strong enough to suppress a muscle-tightening reflex that is protective, so it can be given during labor and delivery to help coordinate exhausted muscles into efficient contractions. Cramp bark combines well with bearberry *(Arctostaphylos uva-ursi)* for bladder infections with painful cramping and frequent urination with little passed. For women's needs generally, cramp bark combines well with black haw *(V. prunifolium)* for painful spasms of the uterus, ovaries, or lower abdomen. In cases of threatened miscarriage, the two together in large doses of tea may allow spasms to subside and normal blood flow to the baby to be maintained. No toxicity is associated with this herb. Because its constituents may be absorbed through the skin, its use in a hot bath helps relax the body, or tincture may be massaged into knotted muscle groups as a liniment.

Tea: 1 to 3 teaspoons (2 to 6 grams) per cup, up to 2 ounces per pint or 3 cups, decocted on low heat for fifteen minutes; take 1 cup three times a day.

Tincture: 1 teaspoon (5 milliliters) three times a day. In instances of extreme need, 1 ounce per dose is immediately effective. In European phytotherapy, up to 6 ounces per week is commonly used to avoid use of suppressive pain medication requiring hospitalization or to reduce the need for allopathic muscle relaxants. As repeated doses or large amounts at a time may be used, a glycerin or nonalcohol preparation is preferred, especially during pregnancy but also when repeated doses or large amounts may be used, such as during periods of heavy menstrual cramps and premenstrual syndrome (PMS).

CURLY DOCK. See YELLOW DOCK

DAMIANA. *Turnera diffusa.* **Part used:** Dried leaf gathered during flowering.

Indications: Damiana, an excellent strengthening remedy for the nervous system, also has an ancient reputation as an aphrodisiac in its native Mexico. It is considered a specific antidepressant where anxiety is complicated by issues of sexuality, including chronic infections of the nervous system related to the reproductive tract, such as herpes. It seems to be strengthening to the libidos of both genders.

Combinations: For people with herpes infections, damiana is often combined with antivirals such as licorice *(Glycyrrhiza glabra)* and St. John's wort *(Hypericum perforatum),* the latter also having an affinity for the nervous system, as well as adaptogens such as Siberian ginseng *(Eleutherococcus senticosus).*

Tea: 1 to 3 teaspoons (2 to 6 grams) dried leaves steeped in 1 cup boiling water, covered, for fifteen minutes; up to 2 ounces per quart, 1 cup one to four times a day.

Tincture: 1 teaspoon (5 milliliters) diluted in 1 cup liquid, one to three times a day. Lower doses provide effective antidepressant effects over time.

DANDELION. *Taraxacum officinale.* **Parts used:** Leaf, root. Leaves are collected during flowering in spring or early summer while they are more tender, less bitter, and less fibrous than later in the year. The root is collected before flowering in the spring for its higher fructose level and its nutrients, which stimulate liver and kidney cleansing. Or the root may be collected after seed has dispersed in the autumn for its higher inulin or starch levels, which make it a good coffee substitute. The root is a short, thick taproot, brown on the outside but cream to white inside.

Indications: Dandelion can be equivalent to certain diuretic prescription drugs but is naturally rich in potassium, which diuretic drugs cause our bodies to lose. Dandelion leaf is given to people experiencing water retention, including swelling of the ankles and generalized puffiness, and it is safe enough to be used by people with a history of damaged kidneys at the dose of 140 milligrams dried herb or its equivalent daily. In healthy patients, use of the leaf extract only shows a slight increase in urination.

Juice from the fresh root and leaf, tea, or tincture of the whole plant is given for reducing congestion of the liver, including portal hypertension associated with cirrhosis (scarring after damage to liver cells), swelling of the tissues caused by liver problems (hepatic edema), hemorrhoids, and varicose veins. The root is less diuretic than the leaf. It assists elimination, helping to clear conditions of the joints, liver, and gallbladder. As a mild bitter tonic, dandelion root stimulates normal hydrochloric acid levels and digestive enzymes, stabilizes blood sugar, and assists bile production and release from the liver and gallbladder to break down dietary fats in the intestines and smooth the way for easier elimination. It is given to prevent gallstones or to treat them long term.

The root is used for chronic skin problems and is given for mild liver toning effects when a congested liver cannot process cyclical hormones, which may lead to imbalances such as premenstrual syndrome (PMS) and estrogen-sensitive fibroids.

Used together, dandelion leaf and root extracts increase cellular metabolism, including circulation of minerals and vitamins to connective tissue that do not receive direct nourishment via the blood vessels. This helps explain its use for arthritis and other joint diseases and as an alterative for improving chronic lack of mobility and function. The root is used to eliminate metabolic toxins such as uric acid, which causes joint pain and gout.

Dandelion also has been given as a tonic for inflammations of the liver including hepatitis, though in the case of infectious hepatitis it may be best combined with stronger antimicrobial herbs such as mountain grape *(Berberis aquifolium)*, or, in serum hepatitis, with other hepatic tonics such as milk thistle *(Silybum marianum)*. In non-A, non-B hepatitis, dandelion is still used but rarely as a single herb; more often it is used in a broader holistic treatment aimed at the possible autoimmune or chronic degenerative processes involved.

Symbolically and literally, dandelion is given to "liverish" or angry, irritable people. It is said that the liver is the seat of the so-called negative emotions that spiritually aware people are not "supposed to" have: fear, envy, anger. Regular use of dandelion allows both emotional and physiocal "static" to clear, perhaps by strengthening the organ that processes toxins and tensions.

Whether used for constipation or PMS, all plant parts of dandelion have been observed to stir up old emotional blocks. If you face these feelings, you can transform them into energy and recycle that energy into creativity.

Used externally, the juice of the plant, including the fresh milky sap, is known as an antimitotic wart remover, though no guarantees can be given for all cases of warts.

Caution: Children love to play with dandelions but can become nauseous from sucking or eating flowers and stems containing fresh milky sap. However, this is not a problem when using dandelion flower wine or any plant part in tea, tincture, or other prepared forms of medicine. Nausea from sucking fresh stems with sap can usually be eased with 2 cups tea containing equal parts of chamomile, marshmallow, and fennel seeds.

Tea: Leaf tea—1 to 2 teaspoons (2 to 4 grams) dried herb per cup; infuse for ten minutes. Use up to 2 ounces per 3 cups; take 1 cup three times a day. Time last doses of day to empty bladder well before bedtime. Root tea—2 to 4 teaspoons (4 to 8 grams) in 3 cups water, simmered fifteen minutes, 1 cup two to three times a day. This can be increased in strength by using up to 2 ounces per pint, 1 cup three times a day.

Tincture: 1 to 2 teaspoons (5 to 10 milliliters) of fresh leaf and/or root juice (if both, use equal parts, preserved with 30 percent alcohol, set for one week, and then strained); take three to six times a day for up to three weeks. Changes after this regimen will suggest whether or not an herbalist's supervision is needed. Leaf tincture—1/2 to 1 teaspoon (2 1/2 to 5 milliliters) two to four times a day, up to 6 ounces per week. Root tincture—1 to 2 teaspoons (5 to 10 milliliters) in water, three times a day, up to 4 ounces per week. Fresh juice may be more effective than excess tea or tincture in achieving strongly diuretic effects in cases of severe water retention, and has been shown since 1911 and as late as 1949 to be safe, though doses of more than 2 tablespoons of juice per day may not ensure the replacement of potassium that dandelion gives at lower therapeutic doses.

DONG QUAI, TANG KWEI. *Angelica sinensis.* **Part used:** Root slices, usually "cured."

Indications: Dong quai has been used to nourish anemic or weak women with long menstrual cycles and congestive dysmenorrhea. In early menopause it can promote the continuing endogenous production of estrogen. Chinese research has shown that if estrogen is low, the phytoestrogens in dong quai act enough like it to help relieve menopausal symptoms while stimulating the body's own estrogen production. If instead there is an excess of estrogen, the phytoestrogens of dong quai bind with estrogen receptor sites, but they are weaker than human or animal estrogen and so have a far weaker physiological effect than estrogen would have. Meanwhile, because the phytoestrogens are competing with estrogen for receptor sites, the excess estrogen in the bloodstream is broken down as it circulates through the liver. This may explain dong quai's apparent "amphoteric," or balancing, effect, which is different depending on the internal environment. Dong quai has been used for reducing hot flashes and certain estrogen-dependent growths; in addition, it has moisturizing effects in cases of vaginal dryness caused by lack of estrogen in menopausal and postmenopausal women. It promotes circulation and general, nonspecific immune resistance. It is usually given between ovulation and day 1 of the menstrual cycle in most premenopausal women or throughout cycles without bleeding in perimenopausal women.

Contraindications: Dong quai can increase blood loss if taken during menstrual bleeding and may be contraindicated in instances of spotting, midcycle bleeding, or flooding, especially of uncertain diagnosis.

Tea: 1 teaspoon (2 grams) of root slice, coarsely crumbled and steeped in 1/4 to 1 cup boiling water in a well-covered container for twenty minutes; 1 cup one to six times a day as needed.

Tincture: 10 drops to 1 teaspoon diluted in 1 cup liquid, one to six times or more as needed each day, especially to assist in managing hot flashes. That may seem a lot, but it isn't if you remember that even the higher daily dose of 6 teaspoons is equal to 2 tablespoons, 30 milliliters, or 1 ounce, taken in increments in the course of the day.

ECHINACEA, also called PURPLE CONEFLOWER. *Echinacea purpurea,* other *Echinacea* species. **Parts used:** All, especially root. Leaves, flowers, and seeds cause a strong (but safe) tingling sensation when chewed well, but the root has the most pronounced effect. There are nine medicinal species, the main ones being *Echinacea purpurea* (purple coneflower), *E. angustifolia* (narrow leaved), *E. pallida* (pale flowered), and *E. tennesiensis*. All four work just fine.

Indications: A nonspecific stimulant to the immune system, echinacea is given in cases of poor or disordered immune response, including the apparent overactivity of autoimmune disorders, hypersensitivities, and allergic reactions. It stimulates the adrenal cortex, partly explaining its use in stress-related immune conditions. In relatively high doses of 3 ounces of tincture per week, echinacea effectively combats viruses by blocking viral attachment to cells while stimulating T-cells, interferon, properdin/complement, and related immune factors. The herb prevents or treats both acute (short-term) infections and chronic infections, including recurrent colds, influenza ("flu"), herpes, and glandular fever. The polyacetylene echinalone from *E. angustifolia,* an insect hormone like those of pyrethrum and feverfew, has antitumor activity. As a biochemical group, the polyacetylenes, also found in other herbs, are proven to be effective against bacteria, including staph (staphylococcus) and strep (streptococcus) as well as fungi. It has been used in holistic approaches to carcinoma (cancer).

Echinacea may be prepared as a water-based tea or an extract of alcohol or glycerin and used internally or externally, but glycerin extracts and tea are not equivalent in strength for fighting infections. Echinacea is safe for internal use during pregnancy, especially as tea; even tincture is infinitely preferable to antibiotics during this tender time.

A hot controversy is raging as to whether it is safe to take this immune herb all the time in case it suppresses the immune system, as antibiotics do. It is usually unnecessary to take echinacea long enough to do this, and no evidence indicates that the whole plant used in the dosages listed below has caused immunity buildup in humans. In my experience, taking it for three or four months when there is a genuine need (serious threat of infection, chronic infection) does not depress the immune system to the degree that it doesn't respond on demand. Nevertheless, it is a waste to take echinacea every day when nothing much is wrong, "just in case." Echinacea works best when it is taken for a period of a few days, weeks, or a few months to treat or prevent infection. Traditionally, it was used frequently and for everything. Research shows that the immuno-stimulating action fades quickly, leaving the natural defenses to take over. For this reason, it is best taken frequently and repeatedly in a crisis.

Combinations: Because echinacea is endangered in the wild from overharvesting, obtain it from reputable companies that grow it organically and use less rather than more. Echinacea synergizes (combines well) with other lymphatic and alterative herbs, so to conserve it, you can use it in mixtures to make the most of small doses or substitute it, depending on the circumstances, with any one or more of the following: yerba santa *(Eriodictyon californica)*, chaparral *(Larrea divericata, L. mexicana)*, yerba mansa *(Anemopsis californica)*, Oregon mountain grape *(Berberis aquifolium)*, wild indigo *(Baptisia tinctoria)*, devil's club *(Oplopanax horridum—* love that name!), hemp agrimony *(Eupatorium cannabinum),* or even humble, hot horseradish *(Armoracia rusticana)*. When in doubt about an alternative herb, ask for a specific recommendation from a practicing herbalist.

Because it is a penetrating antimicrobial for difficult-to-reach places, it combines well with nasturtium as a remedy for pelvic inflammatory disease (PID); in men with prostatitis, it is effective when combined with saw palmetto *(Serenoa serrulata)*.

Note: The higher the quality of the fresh or dried root or any extract, the stronger the tingling or numbing sensation on the tongue. If it doesn't numb the tongue, it is adulterated or is old or of low quality; don't buy it.

Tea: 1/2 teaspoon (1 gram) by infusion, even though roots are usually simmered or decocted. Tea may be as strong as 2 to 3 ounces per pint, and you can take 1 to 10 cups a day.

Tincture: A single dose may range from 15 drops (1 milliliter) up to 2 teaspoons (10 milliliters; 1/3 ounce), diluted in water and taken three times a day may be used for more direct antimicrobial or immune-modulating effects. As little as 2/3 to 1 ounce (20 to 30 milliliters) a week will have preventative effects.

EVENING PRIMROSE. *Oenothera biennis.* **Parts used:** Usually seed; also root and leaf. The oil of the seed is not a volatile oil but a fixed oil, like that pressed from sunflower or other seeds, with the difference that it takes a lot of seed to produce a little oil.

Indications: Research shows that the essential fatty acids of the seed oil have a profound normalizing effect. Evening primrose oil is given for abnormal prostaglandin production and problems with fatty acid synthesis. This has wide applications. It is most commonly used to reduce premenstrual syndrome (PMS), lessen breast tenderness associated with hormonal imbalance, improve menopausal changes, and lower excess blood sugar. It is given for metabolism of healthy fatty acids for overweight people and for metabolic disorders, including diabetes. Native Americans used the root tea for obesity and intestinal pain. It is given for chronic inflammatory conditions, including eczema, hayfever, allergies, asthma, and arthritis. It is especially safe for infants' eczema. Gamma linoleic acid (GLA) is changed in the body to a helpful prostaglandin that seems to lower blood pressure and inhibit platelet aggregation. It helps in multiple sclerosis (MS) because the essential fatty acids protect and repair the myelin sheath surrounding the nerves. In Britain, where it is used as treatment for MS and other autoimmune degeneration involving nerve tissues, the National Health Service pays for prescriptions of evening primrose oil.

Evening primrose oil has also been used as an antidepressant and seems most effective where depression is based in physical problems of hormonal imbalance affecting nerve cells and their function. For this reason, in countries other than America it has been used for hyperactive children.

The root is pulped and rubbed on muscles for strength; in this application it can also speed the healing of bruises. The oil applied directly or in a salve is given to shrink and heal hemorrhoids.

Tea: 1 to 3 capsules of oil (250 milligrams each) one to three times a day. For nervous-system benefits and metabolic disorders the dose is 9 to 10 capsules a day, making it unaffordable to many of the women who need it most. New evidence suggests that lower doses may be effective for PMS in some women. The minimum dose is 2 capsules two times a day.

Whole seed: As an optional supplement, not equivalent to evening primrose oil, 1 to 3 teaspoons (2 to 6 grams) mixed in fruit drinks or "smoothies."

FENNEL. *Foeniculum vulgare.* **Parts used:** Leaf, stem, bulb, seed. The leaves are used in salads, the stems and bulb steamed as a vegetable, and the seeds used to flavor baked breads, stews, and digestive tonics. The fleshy bulb seen in produce sections of grocery stores is from the annual *F. vulgare* 'Azoricum,' or Florence fennel. The seeds are the most concentrated in a volatile oil, which relaxes a stressed digestive system and reduces colicky pains and griping.

Indications: Seed or chopped fennel plant is steeped in water for intestinal cleansing because the disinfecting and warming volatile oil of the herb lessens painful spasms. Seeds are chewed and swallowed with a little water to sweeten the breath. The tea or herb is used as food when there is lack of appetite. Fennel warms and disinfects the digestive tract, with a milder effect on the respiratory linings. The herb promotes the production of breast milk in pregnant or breast-feeding mothers and has a slight estrogen-promoting effect.

Tea: 1/2 to 2 teaspoons (1 to 4 grams) per cup, up to 1/2 to 1 ounce per pint, infused, three cups a day.

Tincture: 1/4 to 1 teaspoon (1 1/2 to 5 milliliters) three times a day.

FEVERFEW. *Chrysanthemum parthenium*, also *Tanacetum parthenium*. **Parts used:** Leaf, flowering top. Herb is best collected and prepared fresh before flowers are fully opened. Only the fresh plant (not the dried herb) is effective.

Indications: Feverfew gradually strengthens the blood vessels in the head, reducing the spasms that trigger migraine headaches. It is clinically used for preventing migraines (one fresh leaf or extract equivalent per day), including menstrual migraines. Although migraine headaches have several causes, feverfew has at least some benefit in all cases. The herb appears to do the most for those able to change their diets and manage stress, both of which can contribute to permanent improvement. Given during migraines, it lessens nausea and vomiting, though it may not help the pain during the episode.

Feverfew lessens muscle spasms partly by keeping calcium in the bloodstream and out of smooth (involuntary) muscle cells. Research indicates that the herb strongly inhibits the formation of prostaglandins, which are involved with our sense of pain, by affecting the way arachidonic acid changes on its way to becoming a prostaglandin. This antiprostaglandin effect also lowers fevers by reducing platelets, which additionally helps thin blood, though this action does not affect healthy blood clotting. In addition, the physiological pathway of feverfew's effects is different from the similar anti-inflammatory effect of salicylate-containing herbs such as willow bark *(Salix alba)*. Feverfew inhibits secretion of serotonin as well as proteins from polymorphonuclear leucocytes, white blood cells that increase in infections and rheumatoid arthritis. Though serotonin is also helpful to mood, interestingly, human clinical trials indicate that feverfew's reduction of this complex substance isn't matched by a worsening of mood. On the contrary, subjects said that even before their pain improved, they had a vague feeling of wellness. Indeed, one of the side effects of using feverfew established now in the scientific literature is "euphoria."

The fresh plant can be made into an aromatic herb vinegar or herb oil, so eating a salad with a homemade dressing containing feverfew every day is one easy way to stay well. The British physicians who took out the patent on the extract following the London Migraine Clinic trials (1982) feel the properties come out well in cold-pressed vegetable oil, though the bitter flavor may not suit all tastebuds.

Feverfew is given for other inflammatory pains of the head or muscular joints. Alhough feverfew can cool down a fever, that is not its main use, nor has that use been researched as well as the others described above.

Contraindications: It is usually considered safe to take feverfew daily for years and years, and people do. However, sensitive people who experience mouth blisters should take a few weeklong breaks if they use the herb longer than six to eight months. It is also too strong in pregnancy, though some women have prevented migraines in the second and third trimester of a healthy term by taking low doses (1 milliliter) after achieving initial advantage over the headaches by other methods.

Combinations: Feverfew combines well with chasteberry *(Vitex agnus-castus)* for menstrual migraines and skullcap *(Scutellaria laterifolia)* for tension migraines.

Tea: Daily dosages range from 50 to 150 milligrams of fresh leaf. For the authentic garden medicine off the stem, try one full, fresh leaf per day for a minimum of twenty days and then increase to two or three leaves a day. After a total of ninety days without migraine or headache, reduce gradually to one-half leaf per day for two months; then a quarter leaf per day for a month; then a quarter leaf every other day for a month. Continue to gradually lower the dose: a quarter leaf every three days, then four, then once a week. The importance of gradual increase and decrease is twofold. First, it helps minimize the blistering or soreness of the tongue that sensitive people experience from the acrid leaves, and smaller doses give mild warnings before this side effect is too uncomfortable. In such cases, switching to freeze-dried herb in capsules is a good alternative. Second, dropping the herb "cold turkey," whether or not it has done the job, may likely result in a merciless rebound headache. When six or more months of this gradual increase and decrease has been successfully completed, one may quit and see how long it takes before the migraines return, if at all. The whole course of treatment may be repeated until the headaches are fewer and farther between each time. Unless dietary triggers and stresses creep back into the person's lifestyle, the migraines should be kept at bay indefinitely.

Capsules: If freeze-dried fresh leaf in capsules are used, take according to directions on packaging or 25 milligrams daily. Some people report that the convenience of capsules doesn't outweigh the uncertainty of their effectiveness. For some they work; for others they don't.

Tincture: 1 teaspoon (5 milliliters) once a day for ninety days, then reduced as outlined above.

Fresh herb vinegar: 1/2 teaspoon twice a day, up to 1 1/2 teaspoons once a day; may be taken diluted in water or other liquid, on salads, or with steamed vegetables.

FLAX. *Linum usitatissimum.* **Parts used:** Whole or freshly crushed seed; sometimes expressed fixed oil.

Indications: Given internally for premenstrual syndrome (PMS), degenerative conditions of nerves and immunity, various conditions of weakness and dryness. Externally used as hot poultice for inflamed boils, as herb plaster over weakened lungs with chronic bronchitis.

Tea: 2 to 12 250-milligram capsules of oil per day, for minimum of six weeks and a maximum of seven years before giving the body a break.

Fresh flax seed oil: 1 teaspoon to 1 tablespoon in a carrier (food, juice) to lubricate intestines. 1-ounce doses of free running oil may act as moisturizing, anti-inflammatory purgative.

GERMAN CHAMOMILE. See CHAMOMILE

GINGER. *Zingiber officinale.* **Part used:** Whole ripened root. In commerce root usually comes peeled and sun-bleached ("white"); sometimes African ginger is unpeeled ("black").

Indications: Ginger is a peripheral-circulation tonic that acts especially well in three areas of capillary beds (tiny blood vessels): the skin, lungs, and gastrointestinal tract. It diffuses warmth through the body from the center outward, so ginger is considered a specific healing agent for brittle capillaries and a tendency to get chills too easily. As a skin capillary treatment it is used for rosacea, the reddened nose of both alcoholics and those with vascular instability. It has been used externally and internally for frostbite. In the lungs its warming action is strongly antimicrobial as well as normalizing where there is excess mucus or dry hacking cough. In the digestive tract ginger has been shown most effective for allaying morning sickness without toxicity in pregnancy. It is also used for travel sickness, nausea generally, and disorders of orientation and motion such as Meniere's disease and vertigo. Especially when used fresh, it reduces microbes on contact in the digestive tract, and it always reduces excess stomach acid and peristaltic spasms, even though it is spicy hot to the taste. It is liver protecting especially when fresh. Ginger is an anticonvulsant that has enormous value in stabilizing blood sugar, when it may be a cofactor for extreme nervous activity and seizures but has limited use in grand mal epilepsy. It helps healthy younger people wake up quickly without coffee or other nerve stimulants.

Combinations: Because it increases circulation, including mild cerebral stimulation, ginger is used as a synergist with ginkgo and other tonic herbs to treat senile atrophy. It lowers high blood cholesterol, making it an excellent choice for daily consumption with garlic *(Allium sativum)* in vegetable dishes. It combines well in lungs with horsetail *(Equisetum arvense)* and other silica-containing herbs specifically toning to connective tissue.

Tea: 1/8 to 1/2 teaspoon (1/4 to 1 gram) per dose, infused (although it is a root, it is not boiled because it contains volatile components) ten to fifteen minutes, up to 1 ounce per pint, 1/2 cup three times a day. Safety and dosage issues have been well established through its long use by humans and confirmed by modern trials.

Fresh root: 1 tablespoon grated or chopped root per cup, infused five minutes well covered; 1/2 cup one to three times a day.

Tincture: 20 drops to 2/3 teaspoon (1 1/2 to 3 milliliters) in water, one to three times a day. Because ginger extracts well, it can be made into a syrup or glycerin extract. *Note:* In cases of sensitive, weak, or older people, start with small doses (5 to 20 drops) of an alcohol-based tincture of fresh root, and use a weekly maximum of 1/2 ounce of a standard alcohol-based tincture of dried root.

GINKGO, also called MAIDENHAIR TREE. *Ginkgo biloba.* **Part used:** Leaf, after turning yellow in fall.

Indications: Ginkgo is used for slowing or reversing memory loss. Its flavonoids have a beneficial action on cardiovascular conditions, especially in improving blood flow to the brain. It helps mood, gently dilates blood vessels, and is considered to be a nerve, heart, and blood vessel tonic. It is remarkably nontoxic and so is used with the elderly and may have value as part of a holistic treatment for people with Alzheimer's. The inner nut is a culinary delicacy used in China for lung problems including tuberculosis. A 24% ginkgolide standardized plant extract inhibits the body's inflammatory response in allergic shock and asthma, and the whole herb has been used as a tonic.

Note: Rarely, with overdoses or self-medication with concentrated standard extracts, there are side effects (dermatitis, diarrhea, vomiting, and irritability). No side effects have been reported with whole plant extracts such as simple tincture or tea.

Tea: 2 to 3 teaspoons (4 to 6 grams) per cup, up to 3 ounces per quart, infused twenty to thirty minutes; take 3 to 4 cups a day. Be aware that the leaf is so light that it is hard to stuff that much in a cup or quart jar; instead, shred the dry leaves in a coffee grinder or blender.

Tincture: 1 teaspoon (5 milliliters) diluted in water, four times a day. Take commercial extract as directed on label, though note that effectiveness varies from brand to brand, and advantages of one over another may not be as advertised.

GINSENG, also called ASIAN or CHINESE GINSENG. *Panax ginseng.* See also AMERICAN GINSENG, SIBERIAN GINSENG. **Part used:** Root. In Asia, it is traditionally cured, turning the root into its distinctive red or deep golden color.

Indications: Ginseng is used to increase physical, mental, emotional, and spiritual strength and integration. It has a stimulating effect on the central nervous system so is given to improve mental alertness and memory.

Ginseng is given to promote higher energy levels with better stability and less agitation. It is given to those with chronic fatigue with or without viral diagnosis as well as to weak, debilitated people. It helps clear shortness of breath with perspiration, anemia, and poor blood circulation and quality. It can lower high blood pressure and stabilize blood sugar. Ginseng increases cellular response to immune challenges including stress. It promotes the functions of the spleen, including the recycling of old red blood cells and the spleen's role in digestion and metabolism. Ginseng also has been shown to promote healthy levels of platelets and to slow the general degeneration associated with aging. How or when it works as an antitumor agent is uncertain; tests with ether extracts on lab cultures of cancer cells show weak activity. But it is known that the phytosterols present in ginseng do not increase growth of tumors and may be a protective synergist with human mechanisms intact in the living person. Ginseng may have a role in nerve repair and growth.

So much has been claimed about the herb, so many warnings arise from pharmacological experiments using isolated constituents on animals, and so many cultural biases against it exist that there is little wonder that its effects are controversial. It is not traditionally given to menopausal women in Asia, perhaps in part because their diets make them less likely to have hot flashes and osteoporosis. But ginseng has good-to-terrific effects when given to women in the West undergoing the Change if their physical symptoms are debilitating and depressing. Ginseng will not make women grow abnormal facial hair or a penis, as has been claimed. Considering that some traditional cultures haven't given women full and equal status, it is no surprise this valuable root has been off limits to women, reserved to keep aging men youthful and to prevent male impotence. Ginseng is a powerful "yang" tonic, meaning that it stimulates several organ functions for an overall energizing effect. The term *yang* does not mean "male," but it does indicate a cultural view of "dynamic activity" as being more masculine than feminine.

Ginseng is especially useful for women of all ages above puberty when they are emotionally stressed, except during pregnancy. It can be used as a crisis tonic for fatigue during late-night cramming for tests, long journeys, or important jobs. Women who have undergone surgical menopause through hysterectomy have used it to regain their vital spark. It has been used at low dose for long-term improvement of women who are passive or submissive, allowing their more assertive energies to be nourished and unfold according to their own right nature. It is best for women who need to increase their estrogen, but not for women with excess estrogen. When in doubt, refer to an herbalist, a doctor of Oriental medicine, or an acupuncturist for more individualized information.

Contraindications: Ginseng is not given to hot, dry people; it may make them dizzy. Women and men who feel tired but have plenty of energy that is not channeled creatively may find that ginseng gives them a headache. Though it lowers blood pressure, it is not recommended for people with extremely high blood pressure because of the variety of factors involved in safely lowering blood pressure. In addition, it is not recommended for people who get nosebleeds easily or women with heavy menstrual bleeding.

Combinations: Ginseng combines well with licorice (*Glycyrrhiza* species) for its antiallergy, immune effects. It combines well with echinacea (*Echinacea* species) and other antimicrobial tonics in chronic immune challenges, as well as in low doses with high doses of hawthorn *(Crataegus oxyacantha)* for aggravated nervous conditions affecting the heart.

Note: Avoid late-night doses if sleeping becomes erratic and mental alertness keeps one up composing lists or conversations or long novels. For sensitive people, the last dose may be timed to occur between midday and mid-afternoon. It can be taken as needed for one to two years but should not be taken every day for longer periods without frequent breaks. Avoid in pregnancy.

Tea: 1/2 to 2 teaspoons (1/2 to 3 grams) per cup, infused thirty minutes or longer. Alternatively, the root may be decocted on low heat in a covered container for fifteen to twenty minutes and left to steep for another fifteen minutes. One cup is taken one to three times a day. The soft pieces at the bottom may be chewed and swallowed to add extra oomph to the dose.

Tincture: 10 to 20 drops (1 to 2 milliliters), up to 1 teaspoon (5 milliliters), in water, one to three times a day.

GUELDER ROSE. See CRAMP BARK

HAWTHORN. *Crataegus oxyacantha, C. laevigata, C. monogyna.* **Parts used:** Flower, leaf, berry. The berry is most common in commerce because it is the most stable in storage, but it is the least potent. The flowers are the most active part, and the leaves are also of greater value than the berry. In phytomedicine a mixture of equal parts is preferred.

Indications: Hawthorn improves cardiac output—the way the heart acts as a pump to push out the right amount of blood in the right rhythm throughout the body and back to the heart. Hawthorn opens coronary arteries to nourish the heart muscle with fresh oxygen-rich blood so that it helps the heart better cope with its workload. It restores correct timing to the heart, usually slowing a rapid heartbeat, but it can also strengthen a weak heart so it safely beats faster. Hawthorn usually lowers high blood pressure, especially a raised diastolic. It raises problematic low blood pressure only when that is due to a weak heart muscle resulting from rheumatic fever or illness; then it brings a low blood pressure up to normal. It has been shown to help arrhythmias within ten minutes of a dose, especially paroxysmal tachycardia. It helps peripheral vessels dilate, bringing better blood flow to all tissues and organs, including the kidneys, which explains its Italian and French use as a diuretic. It is specifically indicated for stroke patients, for use after heart attacks, and for prevention of heart attacks and strokes, especially their recurrence. It is used after bypass operations, for high blood pressure, and for aging. In France and Italy, hawthorn is also used as a sedative for heart conditions with a nervous component, an application consistent with Asian medicine, which considers the heart the house of the spirit and which treats anxiety with heart tonics, not just nerve sedatives. The German ministry of health recommends it for slow heart rate with arrhythmias as well as for rapid, but not dangerously fast, heart rate. In Germany it is also used officially for congestion or oppression in the heart region before use of digitalis is prescribed.

Hawthorn always takes a long time to do its best—six months or longer. In all situations, hawthorn offers several benefits to a damaged or stressed cardiovascular system: It is nontoxic, it is nonaccumulative, it does not cause dependence, and it does not require increased doses.

Hawthorn may be taken as a tea or a fresh or dried herb tincture; the berries may be made into syrups and jams or soaked and baked into bread. In England, the elderly sometimes still get hawthorn and rosehip jam for presents from the young, or make their own "haws elixir" soaked in brandy, eating two or three berries a day each winter.

Note: Hawthorn synergizes with other herbs and other heart medications. Since 1938 hawthorn has been known as a nontoxic heart remedy that synergizes with drugs to reduce dosages of medication by 30 to 80 percent. For this reason, when hawthorn is used along with digitalis drugs, a health-care provider must monitor the person's improvements so that the drug dose may be reduced according to the heart's changing needs.

Contraindications: Hawthorn is contraindicated in high doses for people with atrial fibrillation, at least for prolonged periods (several months). Hawthorn may also be contraindicated in severe low blood pressure if that is due to problems with the heart valves rather than the heart muscle and vessels. In these cases, the dosage is 1/2 ounce flower, leaf, and berry in equal parts infused for twenty minutes in 2 cups water, or 15 drops tincture in water twice a day.

Combinations: An official German heart tonic is hawthorn, lavender, and lemon balm as a tea, tincture, or cordial. Hawthorn also combines well with passion flower for this effect.

Tea: 1/2 to 1 teaspoon (1 to 2 grams) per cup, three times a day. Infuse flowers and leaves; simmer or decoct berries. Small doses range from 1 to 5 tablespoons of tea per day. A standard dose is 1 ounce per pint, 1 cup three times a day. If flowers, leaves, and berries are mixed together, use 1 ounce to 1 quart water and infuse or steep longer (twenty to thirty minutes) rather than decocting.

Tincture: Minimum of 15 drops twice a day; standard range is 1/4 to 1/2 teaspoon (12 drops or 2 1/2 milliliters) three times a day. The herb can be taken safely in larger amounts according to need; however, a health-care provider should monitor progress, such as improvements in blood pressure, to avoid overmedication with prescription drugs.

HIBISCUS. *Hibiscus sabdariffa.* **Part used:** Flower.

Indications: Used for reducing inflammations, fevers, and sweats; improves flavor of other preparations.

Note: This sweet-sour tonic is a member of the Malva family. It is not interchangeable with the ornamental shrub hibiscus, which is often hybridized and/or sprayed.

Tea: 1 to 2 teaspoons (2 to 4 grams) per cup, up to 2 ounces per pint, infused; drink 1/2 cup three times a day.

Tincture: 1 teaspoon (5 milliliters) diluted in water, one to eight times a day as desired.

HIGHBUSH CRANBERRY. See CRAMPBARK

HORSETAIL, also called SHAVEGRASS. *Equisetum arvense.* **Parts used:** Stem and branches (needles) collected in springtime or early summer while still bright green, before full height is reached. Later in summer the herb is drier or "bristly" to the touch, taller, and a dull green to gray or even pale brown.

Indications: Horsetail's high silicic acid content makes it an astringent for the reproductive and urinary systems as well as a nutritive for bones, joints, and connective tissue; it also speeds the healing of wounds. Horsetail is primarily given for urinary discharges, infections, inflammations, and, in men, for benign enlargement of the prostate. Used in excess, it can irritate damaged kidneys, but in smaller amounts, as noted below, its toning effect is also useful for urinary incontinence. As a remedy that nourishes connective tissue, it is indicated for rheumatic pains as well as inflammation of tendons and ligaments. In this use, it is used internally and as an addition to hot baths (steep 4 ounces of horsetail in 2 pints of water for one hour; strain and add tea to bath). The tea or extract used externally works well on wounds. There is some suggestion that taking extra B-complex foods (whole grains, green leafy vegetables) with horsetail is helpful for relieving joint pain, nourishing bones, and healing wounds.

Combinations: In the genito-urinary system, it combines well with marshmallow *(Althaea officinalis)*, shepherd's purse *(Capsella bursa-pastoris),* or yarrow *(Achillea millefolium).* For nourishing connective tissue, you can combine horsetail with nervines such as wild oats *(Avena sativa)* and St. John's wort *(Hypericum perforatum).* For menopausal changes to skin, hair, bones, and connective tissue, it combines well with reproductive hormonal remedies such as chasteberry *(Vitex agnus-castus)*, black cohosh *(Cimicifuga racemosa)*, angelica *(Angelica archangelica)*, and dong quai *(A. sinensis)*. For clearing respiratory conditions, it works well with licorice *(Glycyrrhiza glabra)*. For internal bleeding it works well with shepherd's purse *(Capsella bursa-pastoris)*.

Tea: 2 teaspoons (4 grams) dry herb steeped in 1 cup boiling water for twenty minutes, up to 1 ounce per pint to three cups; take 1 cup three times a day.

Tincture: 1 teaspoon (5 milliliters), diluted in 1 cup water or other liquid, three times a day.

JAMAICAN SARSAPARILLA. See SARSAPARILLA

LADY'S MANTLE, LADIES MANTLE. *Alchemilla vulgaris.* **Part used:** Flowering herb. Good-quality herb is hard to find, so many students of healing plants have forgotten this helpful plant.

Indications: Problems of imbalance in female reproductive systems and diseases of small blood vessels. Lady's mantle is perhaps the best astringent for reproductive bleeding of a known cause, such as heavy periods and fibroids, in which case it combines well with shepherd's purse *(Capsella bursa-pastoris)*. It is specific for improving poor uterine tone and relieving heavy bleeding, menopausal hot flashes, and vaginitis. It is also indicated for hardening of the arteries and external and internal bruising and wounds. Fresh leaves have been used on *Herpes zoster* (fever blisters and canker sores of the mouth) and other mucous membrane inflammations such as those accompanying pruritus (vaginal itching) and leucorrhea (white discharge). It combines well in equal parts with motherwort *(Leonurus cardiaca)* and chasteberry *(Vitex agnus-castus)* for hot flashes. No toxicity is known; used as directed.

Tea: Liberal amounts of tea are commonly used, especially in instances of overweight with an endocrine cause, such as in menopausal weight gain. To prepare an infusion, boil the standard dose of 1/2 to 1 teaspoon (2 to 4 grams) per cup, or 1/2 to 1 ounce per pint, for one to two minutes; then steep another ten minutes. This will extract all the tannins for stronger astringent action.

Tincture: 1/2 to 1 teaspoon (2 to 5 milliliters) three times a day, up to 3 ounces per week.

LAVENDER. *Lavandula officinalis, L. vera, L. spica.* **Parts used:** Flower, essential oil.

Indications: Lavender is given internally for tension, high blood pressure, and nervous headaches. It is commonly used as emergency treatment for headaches and stiff muscles of head and shoulders (massage a few drops of essential oil into temples, forehead, back of neck, and shoulders). In any form, it is also given for chronic complaints of nervousness to reestablish healthy nerve function rather than to sedate. The warming, relaxing effects of this cleansing herb make it useful for cramps and digestive upsets (diarrhea, gas, sour stomach, constipation). A drop of volatile oil on a handkerchief or in a small vial kept in the pocket can be inhaled several times a day as needed for depression mixed with anxiety, dizziness, vertigo, and headache.

The other main use of lavender is as an antiseptic. Tea or extract is used as a wash externally or as an internal cleansing agent for infections and poor elimination of metabolic toxins or high blood fats. The essential or volatile oil is used externally on wounds, bruises, or deep punctures including insect stings.

An important thing to know is that lavender tea does not taste as great as it sounds: it is bitter and astringent. Nevertheless, it is effective and can be combined as a tea with other delicious herbs if only a little is used. When glycerin is used as the liquid for extraction, rather than alcohol or water, the herb's exquisite fragrance comes through with less soapy, bitter astringency; in addition, this method reduces the potential problem of lavender's tannins binding with another herb's alkaloids in a compound of herb extracts.

Combinations: For circulatory conditions lavender combines well with linden flower *(Tilia europaea, T. platyphyllos)*, yarrow *(Achillea millefolium)*, or rosemary *(Rosmarinus officinalis)*. Lavender relaxes and opens up arteries as it stimulates circulation, while rosemary constricts overdilated arteries, the volatile oils of both stimulating better flow of blood around the body. In addition, rosemary adds its characteristic effect of awakening alertness and memory. The two herbs—relaxing and stimulating—don't cancel each other out but find a happy medium when used together. For nervous conditions lavender combines with vervain *(Verbena officinalis)*, motherwort *(Leonurus cardiaca)*, or skullcap *(Scutellaria laterifolia)*. It is safely used during pregnancy.

Tea: 1 to 2 1/2 teaspoons (2 to 5 grams) per cup, 1 ounce per pint, infused ten minutes in a closed container; take 1 cup three times a day (it tastes awful, so you may want to add honey).

Tincture: 1/2 to 1 teaspoon (2 1/2 to 5 milliliters) in water, three times a week (up to 3 ounces per week). Glycerin extract is given at the same dosage as for tincture and has a lovely taste.

Essential oil: Use essential oil externally, or drink 1 drop stirred in one 8-ounce cup of juice to settle the nausea of migraine. Add a few drops of essential oil to a bath or steam inhalation for cleansing the skin or reducing tension.

Facial steams of essential oil may be used by teenagers, moms, or women going through or past the Change for acne and cysts associated with hormonal changes or stress. Lavender herb or essential oil in a facial steam is also soothing to the nerves and used for tension headaches, infected sinuses, and irritations of upper respiratory passages. Place 1 to 3 drops of essential oil in a large bowl or container of just-boiled water; place face 10 or so inches above steam; cover head and bowl of lavender water with a large towel; breathe in for ten to fifteen minutes. Repeat every night for one week; then reduce only as needed.

LEMON BALM. *Melissa officinalis.* **Part used:** Leaf. Lemon balm is one of the most fragile of volatile oil-containing herbs, so the leaves are picked in the morning before the heat of the day rises and dried quickly by dehumidification. Unbroken leaves last in storage for four to six months in airtight containers, so gardeners plan for two harvests a year of this quick-growing perennial. When buying herb for tea, crumble a dried leaf to be sure it smells minty and lemony.

Indications: Lemon balm is given for depressive illness or restlessness. The oils and tannins it contains make it a useful herb for tension migraines, especially when digestive problems are also present. Lemon balm is given for nervous indigestion of all descriptions and for poor circulation (feeling either too hot or too cold). Lemon balm also sweetens a nervous, acid stomach. It is antiviral, especially drunk as a tea, against *Herpes simplex.* The herb and the volatile or essential oil used in aromatherapy are given for depression, nervousness, insomnia, and tension headaches.

Note: The herb tea is enjoyed by many as a beverage during early pregnancy to allay morning sickness. However, for some women and all pregnant women, individual taste and smell are peculiarly unpredictable, so if it doesn't sit well with you, choose any of the many other herbs with similar actions.

Combinations: Lemon balm combines well with peppermint *(Mentha piperita)*, ginger root *(Zingiber* species), and raspberry leaf *(Rubus idaeus)* for indigestion or morning sickness; and with motherwort *(Leonurus cardiaca)* for agitated nerves and poor circulation. For a quick calming effect, combine it with angelica root, lemon peel, cinnamon, and honey or one's choice of natural sweetener (2 to 3 drops on the tongue as needed).

Tea: 1 to 2 teaspoons (2 to 4 grams) per cup, 1/2 to 1 ounce per pint, infused, 1 cup three times a day.

Tincture: 1/2 to 1 teaspoon (2 1/2 to 5 milliliters) diluted in water, one to four times a day.

LEMON GRASS. *Cymbopogon citratus.* **Parts used:** Leaf, essential oil for external use.

Indications: Used for balancing uneven skin tone, both oily and dry areas, through improved circulation, digestion, liver, and lymphatic functions.

Tea: 1 to 2 teaspoons per cup (2 to 4 grams), up to 2 ounces per pint, infused; take 1 cup three times a day.

Tincture: 1 teaspoon (5 milliliters) diluted in water, one to eight times a day as desired.

LEMON VERBENA. *Lippia citriodora*, also *Aloysia triphylla*. **Note:** Not to be confused with *Verbena officinalis* (vervain, a bitter-tasting tonic). **Part used:** Leaf.

Indications: Used for flavoring and to reduce heat, bloating, gas, and indigestion.

Tea: 1 to 2 teaspoons (2 to 4 grams) per cup, up to 2 ounces per pint, infused; take 1 cup three times a day.

Tincture: 1 teaspoon (5 milliliters) diluted in water, one to eight times a day as desired.

LICORICE, LIQUORICE. *Glycyrrhiza glabra*. **Parts used:** Dried root collected in late autumn, thoroughly cleaned, sliced thin, and dried. Leaf is also used.

Indications: Licorice's many powerful constituents make it effective in increasing the body's secretion of bile while moistening intestinal contents for better elimination from the digestive tract. It is soothing and relaxing to smooth muscle in the gastrointestinal tract on contact. Licorice gets into a painful, contracted, tight, wounded digestive tract and coats over the raw place, relaxes the clenched-up involuntary muscles, and acts as a local anti-inflammatory. The flavonoids it contains are probably the part that gives us the muscle-relaxing effect for intestinal colic or spasm. Licorice is even more renowned as a healing agent for ulcers, both gastric and duodenal. It is widely used as an herb to improve the flavor of herbal formulas, especially in cough and lung combinations, where its saponins help clear respiratory congestion. Licorice root is indicated for chronic coughs, bronchial congestion, and bronchitis as a soothing decongestant. It also synergizes with adrenal gland tonics, especially to treat hypoglycemia or low blood sugar. Perhaps surprisingly, it is indicated in small amounts as a way to reduce sugar cravings and safely increase sweetness for people with diabetes. Licorice also decreases blood cholesterol. In small amounts combined with modifying herbs specific to the individual, licorice has been used safely long term (years) by clients with chronic inflammatory disease. It is indicated for tissue damage from the mouth all the way down to the small intestine. Research has shown it to decrease high testosterone levels in women with ovarian cysts and to increase their fertility. In 1985 the *Journal of Pharmacological Sciences* reported its effectiveness against *Streptococcus mutans,* plaque formation, and dental caries. In Chinese medicine it is considered harmonizing in complex formulas. Externally the herbal preparation is used as an anti-inflammatory, antiviral, demulcent vulnerary for skin wounds and eye inflammations.

Contraindications: The whole herb, traditionally recommended by herbalists, has not been associated with the side effects of excess aldosterone (edema, heart failure) or low potassium (weakness) that can occur with eating large quantities of licorice candy or high doses of concentrated extracts continually taken for extended periods. Licorice can have these potentially harmful side effects in people who have low renin (a hormone affecting blood pressure), hypokalemia (low blood potassium), hypertension (high blood pressure, especially with water retention or edema), or a history of renal (kidney) or cardiac (heart) failure. A study of healthy subjects eating 3 ounces of licorice candy every day for a few weeks showed that some had temporary edema and low potassium, and a few had temporarily elevated blood pressure. A study in Italy compared the potassium effects from licorice to those of steroidal nasal sprays, finding them more or less equal. Glycyrrhizin, a chemical in licorice, is unsafe at doses of 0.5 gram, equivalent to 5 grams (5,000 milligrams) of herb per day. Elderly persons are especially helped by conservative dosage for a number of reasons. First, because metabolism often is slower as we age, the half-life of the herb, as with any substance, is longer in the elderly, so its effects on potassium and water retention are greater. Second, older people are more likely to use digitalis or related heart drugs and/or conventional diuretics that cause one to lose potassium, which licorice may do as well. In addition, an individual with arthritis may be taking steroidal anti-inflammatories that may add to the adrenal effects of licorice, possibly leading in time to increased aldosterone, water retention, edema, and higher blood pressure.

Combinations: For chronic digestive inflammation, licorice combines well with peppermint *(Mentha piperita)*, dandelion root *(Taraxacum officinale)*, and marshmallow *(Althaea officinale)*. For stimulating endocrine balance, it combines well with wild yam *(Dioscorea villosa)* and Siberian ginseng *(Eleutherococcus senticosus)*. For the cardiovascular system, it combines well with hawthorn (*Crataegus* species) and reishi *(Ganoderma lucidum)*.

Tea: A safe and effective dose of the herb is 1 teaspoon (2 grams) per cup. Use up to 3 ounces per quart of water, infused (though it's a root). Take 1 cup one to three times a day. If sensitive, use as little as 50 to 100 milligrams of the dried root decocted in a cup of tea taken three times a day.

Tincture: 1/2 to 1 teaspoon (2 1/2 to 5 milliliters) diluted in water three times a day.

LIME BLOSSOM. See LINDEN

LINDEN, also called LIME BLOSSOM. *Tilia europea, T. cordata,* or *T. platyphylla.* **Part used:** Dried flower, gathered after flowering in midsummer, dried carefully in the shade.

Indications: Linden is well known as a relaxing remedy for nervous tension at all ages. It is reputed to prevent hardening of the arteries and high blood pressure by relaxing constricted blood vessels; it also strengthens blood vessels. It is considered to be a specific treatment for raised blood pressure associated with arteriosclerosis and nervous tension. It initially increases peripheral circulation to fingers and toes, helping the evaporation of body heat, and then stabilizes blood vessels and body temperature. Its combined diaphoretic and relaxing effects explain its use in feverish colds and flus.

Combinations: In hypertension it is used with hops or hawthorn; for colds and flus it is used with elder, peppermint, yarrow, or echinacea.

Tea: 1 to 3 teaspoons (2 to 6 grams) dried flowers infused or steeped in 1 cup boiling water, covered, for ten minutes. This mild dose may be increased up to 2 ounces per 3 to 4 cups for stronger effects. Take 1 cup three times a day.

Tincture: 1/2 to 1 teaspoon (2 1/2 to 5 milliliters) three times a day.

LIQUORICE. See LICORICE

MARSHMALLOW. *Althaea officinalis.* **Parts used:** Leaf, root, flowers. For best mucilage, always pick leaves in early summer before flowers are formed, and harvest roots in winter, from marshes or wet depressions in the garden.

Indications: Marshmallow soothes, cools, and moisturizes any dry, irritated surface inside or outside the body. Marshmallow is given to people with dry skin, constipation, or "too little water," as in prolonged fevers, hot flashes, night sweats, or dehydration. Marshmallow is used for smoker's hack, hoarseness, nonproductive coughs, heartburn, hiatal hernia, gastric and duodenal ulcers, malnutrition, overeating, constipation with or without infection, cystitis, and skin burns. The root and leaf extract well in tea, cold infusions, extracts, or syrups. Any part of the mallow can be used to protect stomach linings from inflammation and help rebuild the linings of the digestive system after damage. Its other uses, for kidney and urinary complaints, rely on a combination of both root and flowers for the best moistening, anti-inflammatory action and the added presence of volatile oils in its flowers, which inhibit some germs. On skin, a mash of leaves lessens the pain of bee stings, burns, and traumatic wounds. The roots are used the same way.

Combinations: Marshmallow mixes well with equal parts of bearberry and yarrow for cystitis but should be used by itself or with corn silk *(Zea mays)* for cystitis occurring during pregnancy.

Tea: 1/2 to 3 teaspoons (1 to 6 grams) per cup, infused; use 1/2 to 2 ounces per quart. Take 1 cup three times a day. The hot tea will be thinner than the cold infusion so may be taken more frequently or made stronger; the cold infusion requires less herb.

Tincture: 1/2 teaspoon tincture or up to 6 tablespoons of syrup as needed, up to 8 ounces total per week.

MEADOWSWEET. *Filipendula ulmaria.* Formerly *Spirea ulmaria*, the plant gave its name (a-spirin) to the anti-inflammatory salicylates also found in willow bark (*Salix* species). **Part used:** Flowering herb.

Indications: Meadowsweet is given wherever there is acidity, inflammation, or pain, with or without infection. It is astringent and healing for all discharges, including diarrhea and more chronic digestive problems such as "acid stomach."

In an alkaline pH of the digestive tract, the sodium salicylate it contains is absorbed into circulation and has pain-reducing properties. It is specific for arthritic joint pain. In chronic inflammations of the stomach or intestines, the acidic pH causes the sodium salicylate to form free salicylic acid, where it can act as a strong local anti-inflammatory and antiseptic by destroying bacterial cell proteins. Meadowsweet has traditionally been used to treat stomach ulcers.

Meadowsweet reduces fevers by suppressing the sympathetic temperature regulation center. While the herb is not usually strong enough to suppress a high fever, with other antimicrobials or febrifuges it can help manage a fever in a temperature range comfortable to the human host but incapacitating to the invading germs.

In high amounts (1 to 2 ounces per quart or 1/2 ounce tincture) meadowsweet is a disinfectant for the digestive tract. It is specific for peptic ulcers, hiatal hernia, heartburn, or tendency to excess acidity. In very high amounts (3 ounces per quart or 2 ounces tincture diluted in water per day), meadowsweet will help cleanse an inflamed or infected urinary system and is given for chronic cystitis. It is used liberally in nonalcoholic forms (water-based tea or glycerin tinctures) for gout and kidney stones.

Combinations: Meadowsweet combines with feverfew *(Chrysanthemum parthenium)* for migraines. It combines well with horsetail *(Equisetum arvense)* for tissue healing and for all forms of arthritis.

Tea: The aspirinlike constituents are dilute in their natural, herbal form. One can make a regular 2–4 gram or 2-teaspoon (2-to-4-gram) cup of tea, strain out the herb, and use the tea to steep a new batch of dried herb. This doubles the strength without increasing the amount of tea one needs to take. Infuse 1 to 2 ounces per quart; take 1 cup three to four times a day.

Tincture: 1/2 to 1 teaspoon (2 1/2 to 5 milliliters) three times a day.

MOTHERWORT. *Leonurus cardiaca.* **Parts used:** Leaf, flower, collected before full flowering in early summer, dried in shade.

Indications: This bitter-tasting, heart-strengthening herb lessens anxiety, especially palpitations of the heart, justifying its scientific name, *cardiaca*. It is given for tension in pregnancy, premenstrual sydrome (PMS) with delayed menses, and hot flashes of the Change. It is especially useful for hot flashes associated with nervous tension as the primary trigger, accompanied by palpitations of the heart. Motherwort has been considered a specific treatment for all conditions of hormonal imbalance and nervous tension. This may explain why it is considered good for all mothers, and it has been given to menopausal women and their teenage daughters to achieve a more serene household.

Motherwort is also used to improve circulation, lower blood lipids, and reduce platelet aggregation. It is given for nerve pain and sensitive or painful skin as in herpes or shingles. Motherwort may help an overactive thyroid but does not depress normal thyroid function.

Combinations: For hot flashes, it combines well with dong quai *(Angelica sinensis)* and sage *(Salvia officinalis)*. For hyperthyroidism, it combines well with bugleweed, also called gypsywort *(Lycopus virginicus)*, not to be confused with bugle *(Ajuga reptans)*.

Note: During pregnancy limit motherwort to three weeks at the doses below or take longer in half doses. The bitter flavor is part of the hormone-balancing property of motherwort; in moderation, the herb is extremely helpful for stress. However, too much for too long may interfere with a sensitive pregnant woman's own internal balance.

Tea: 1 to 2 teaspoons (2 to 4 grams) per cup, or 1/2 teaspoon (1 gram) leaves and flower buds steeped in 1 cup water for ten minutes (very mild), up to 1 ounce per pint. Take 1 cup three times a day, or more often in 1/2-cup doses as needed.

Tincture: 10 drops to 3/4 teaspoon (1 to 4 milliliters) or diluted in 1 cup liquid, three times a day. Take more often as needed in 1/2 cup of water, herb tea, or juice, especially for palpitations and hot flashes, rapid pulse, high blood pressure, or just changing a bad state of nerves.

MUGWORT. *Artemisia vulgaris.* **Part used:** Flowering herb.

Indications: Used to stimulate bodily process of menses if delayed by exhaustion, illness, or anorexia. It can be used for nausea, vomiting, and threadworm or roundworm infestation.

Note: Not to be used in pregnancy. The taste is bitter, but only small doses are needed for the indications given above.

Tea: 1/4 to 1 teaspoon (1/2 to 2 grams) per cup, 1/2 cup three times a day thirty minutes before meals.

Tincture: 1/2 teaspoon (2 1/2 milliliters) diluted in water, three times a day, before meals.

NETTLE, also called STINGING NETTLE. *Urtica dioica.* **Parts used:** Usually leaf, also seed. As soon as the herb has been cut and dried, then heated and soaked in water (prepared as a tea or tincture), the needlelike hairs of the herb and the stinging plant acids they contain decompose nicely and lose their sting. Occasionally freshly dried whole nettle leaf and stem may give a temporary tingling redness to hands during preparation and handling, a pleasant sign of potent herb.

Indications: Nettle is used for rebuilding blood in anemic people, especially those with iron deficiency or a history of blood loss such as that occurring with menopausal flooding. This stinging plant has been used externally and internally to stop bleeding, especially uterine bleeding, including during pregnancy for spotting or threatened miscarriage. In later stages of pregnancy or breast-feeding it is a galactagogue and stabilizing blood tonic for blood sugar levels and energy. It is used to normalize the quality of the blood rather than its volume or pressure, and it can be used with other hypotensive or cardiovascular tonic combinations. In arthritis and other inflammatory conditions, nettle stimulates circulation to peripheral and weight-bearing joints, eventually toning connective tissues for greater mobility with less pain. It is also given for improving kidney excretion of metabolic wastes, particularly uric acid, making it specific for gout. Nettle is a universal fortifier for those women who could use the protective and defensive qualities of the herb in symbolic and physiological dimensions.

The astringency of nettle leaf is not constipating, so it can be given for gastric or intestinal ulcers, with or without hemorrhaging, and for coughing up blood— *but* you must consult a health-care provider for diagnosis of these potentially serious conditions before herbal treatment.

Caution: This plant is not toxic in the sense that it is poisonous, but there are reports that long-term, heavy use of nettle, usually too much concentrated tincture, brings a warning sign of slightly scratchy sensations on urination. I have never seen this occur in practice, but students report that they have done it to themselves. For best effects long term, tea is preferred. If you experience any irritation, simply reduce the dose, combine nettle with demulcent diuretics such as marshmallow *(Althaea officinalis)*, or skip it altogether for a while.

Tea: 1 1/2 to 3 teaspoons (3 to 6 grams) per cup, up to 2 ounces per pint or quart, infused fifteen minutes. Take 1 cup three times a day.

Fresh juice: Dose of fresh juice, called a "succus": 1 teaspoon to 1 tablespoon, three times a day. Juice may be preserved for use all year with 30 percent alcohol by volume (3 ounces pure alcohol to 7 ounces juice for 10 ounces total preserved succus) or 60 percent glycerin (6 ounces pure glycerin to 4 ounces fresh juice for 10 ounces glycerin succus).

Tincture: 1 to 2 teaspoons (5 to 10 milliliters) in water, three times a day or more.

OATS, OATSTRAW. See WILD OATS

ORANGE. *Citrus aurantium.* **Parts used:** Peel, oil, juice, fruit.

Indications: Orange is used for aroma and flavor and for aiding the digestion of less pleasant tasting remedies. The juice and fruit provide vitamin C.

Tea: 1/2 to 2 teaspoons (1 to 4 grams) per cup, up to 2 ounces per pint, infused; 1/2 cup three times a day.

Tincture: 1 teaspoon (5 milliliters) diluted in water; take one to eight times a day as desired.

PARA TODO. See SUMA

PARTRIDGE BERRY. *Mitchella repens*. **Parts used:** Dried leaf and stem.

Indications: A nourishing and safe remedy for women from puberty through menopause, including during pregnancy and lactation, especially where there is a history of difficult pregnancy or a weak reproductive system. In cases of chronic weakness or disease, it needs to be taken for four to eight weeks before results may be seen.

Partridge berry is a specific treatment for uterine hemorrhage, and therefore it is indicated in menopausal flooding as well as heavy uterine blood loss of any kind after diagnosis by a health-care provider. Partridge berry may also relieve painful periods.

Tea: 1 teaspoon (2 grams) dried herb per cup, up to 1 ounce per pint, steeped in boiling water, covered, for ten minutes. Take 1 cup three times a day. In pregnancy, use only as needed, limiting dose to 1 cup of tea a day for two to four weeks.

Tincture: 1 to 4 teaspoons (5 to 20 milliliters) diluted in 1 cup water. Take in higher doses (2 to 4 teaspoons) every twenty minutes until excess bleeding slows or stops.

PASSION FLOWER, PASSIONFLOWER. *Passiflora incarnata, P. edulis*. **Parts used:** Leaf, flower, whole plant.

Indications: Extracts have been shown to lower high blood pressure and rapid heartbeat. Passion flower's antispasmodic and anti-inflammatory effects make it a useful treatment for shock and pain, including headache. It is given for insomnia, especially when it is caused by pain. It is given as a nervine tonic for epilepsy. It also reduces premenstrual syndrome (PMS) and mood swings related to menopause.

Note: Passion flower is not an addictive narcotic, and no evidence of toxicity is associated with its use. It has been used instead of synthetic pain relievers during pregnancy with no reported side effects. As it acts on the central nervous system, however, it is not to be used long term in pregnancy and is usually given in conservative doses for seven to ten days. As with most powerful herbs, start with small amounts in pregnancy and repeat until it is effective, as pain thresholds differ greatly among individuals.

Tea: 1/2 to 2 1/2 teaspoons (1 to 5 grams) per cup, up to 2 ounces per 3 cups. Take 1 cup every hour for severe pain; to generally reduce pain or tension, take 1 cup two to three times a day.

Tincture: 10 drops to 1 teaspoon (1 to 5 milliliters) in water every hour as needed for quick relief, or three times a day for general benefits.

PEPPERMINT. *Mentha piperita*. **Parts used:** Leaf, flowering top, essential or volatile oil.

Indications: The flowering tops and leaves are used for indigestion, colic, and irritation of the entire digestive tract. Peppermint settles an overfull or sour stomach; it reduces intestinal bloating by assisting in the elimination of gas, relaxing intestinal spasms, and encouraging helpful intestinal flora to combat bacteria that create extra gas. Peppermint tea, extract, or essential oil can ease hiccups and pressure against the diaphragm. It is also useful as an oral disinfectant for spongy or sore gums.

Tea: 1 to 2 teaspoons (2 to 4 grams) per cup; 1/2 to 1 ounce per pint, 1 cup three times a day.

Tincture: 1/2 to 1 teaspoon (2 1/2 to 5 milliliters) three times a day.

Essential oil: 1 drop in 1 quart water, well shaken; take sips or 1/2 cup as needed.

POT MARIGOLD. See CALENDULA

PURPLE CONEFLOWER. See ECHINACEA

RASPBERRY LEAF. *Rubus idaeus.* **Parts used:** Leaf, flower, berry. For medicinal purposes the leaf is used the most. Raspberry is often given during pregnancy, when alcohol is best avoided, so it is usually taken as a tea. In menopause it may be taken in any form of preparation. Dried flowers may be added to leaf tea; fresh berries provide vitamin C and nutritive properties.

Indications: This herb is known to be a safe, reliable tea for strengthening pregnant women, but it is used by women at other times as well. The leaves have an astringent (toning) effect on the reproductive system and help stimulate normal function. The herb is given to young girls beginning menstrual cycles or experiencing cramps, mothers preparing for a new pregnancy, and menopausal women wishing to prevent loss of tone with age. Raspberry's astringent tannins and nourishing minerals make it especially helpful in painful, prolonged, or heavy menstrual bleeding, though symptoms that do not clear in a few (three) cycles with herbs ought to be assessed by a health professional. Raspberry leaf is used for uterine fibroids. In addition, the minerals in raspberry make it a useful nutritive in cases of dehydration, imbalance of salts, and exhaustion. Though raspberry ensures supplies of rich mother's milk in pregnancy, the herb lessens breast tenderness.

Tea: 1 to 2 1/2 teaspoons (2 to 5 grams) per cup, 1/4 ounce up to 2 ounces per pint, infused for ten to fifteen minutes; take 1 cup two to three times a day. It can be made as strong as you like, but it should have a pleasant taste.

Tincture: 1 teaspoon (5 milliliters) diluted in water; take one to three times a day.

RED CLOVER. *Trifolium pratense.* **Part used:** Freshly dried flower head. Poor commercial samples contain a high proportion of leaves and brown flowers with little or no odor or taste; picked or stored incorrectly, they may contain such different levels of constituents that they cannot be relied upon for effective cleansing.

Indications: As an alterative, red clover is one of the best remedies for childhood eczema or psoriasis. Red clover is a relaxing nervine that settles restlessness in nervous adults but is mild enough for children. It is specific for spasmodic coughing, bronchitis, and asthma in high-strung or sensitive people. It is used to bring on normal menses. Red clover tea is generally regarded as safe to use for promoting fertility as well as during pregnancy and breast-feeding.

Like many other pea family herbs, red clover has some estrogenic plant sterols. It has been given as part of a holistic treatment for breast tumors and fibroids, both associated with excess estrogen, because the herbal version competes with excess estrogen, allowing the body to come into balance.

As an antineoplastic (anticancer) herb, red clover has a widespread and long historical use in folk traditions. It has been used for women's reproductive cancer. One way to prepare it for external use is to fill a crock pot with fresh clover flowers, cover them with cold water and a lid, and turn to low temperature for one to two days or until water is reduced by half. Press out liquid, discard herb, and return liquid to the cleaned crockpot without lid for another two to three days or until the volume has been reduced to a black tar. Stir this with *one* of the following: castor oil, glycerin, or lanolin (avoid if allergic). Apply this sticky paste in liberal coats over lumps. Cover with cotton gauze or a soft, clean cloth; leave on one to two days or until the paste is mostly caked or unevenly dried; then remove most of herb paste by gently sponging warm water over area. Reapply a fresh coat of paste and cover. This treatment is said to be best for reducing growths near the surface and has been used for benign breast lumps, lipomas, or malignant growths, including cancerous skin lesions, though no claims about its anticancer use can be made here.

If you follow this procedure, drink 1 quart of red clover tea twice a day, up to 3 ounces dried or 5 ounces fresh flowers per quart. Some sources say that any estrogenic herb is unsafe in estrogen-dependent cancers, but further clarification is needed to differentiate between isolated estrogens tested on lab animals and research on humans using red clover.

Red clover is generally considered safe and nontoxic in government and medical registers of herbal medicine. However, these amounts (3 to 5 ounces dried herb per quart twice a day) are not recommended for general therapeutic benefits; nor is this amount recommended during pregnancy. Safer, lower doses for general benefit are listed below.

Because chronic, degenerative diseases require large quantities of herb, and because commercial red clover is often of low quality, grow your own healing patch of organic red clover lawn or buy from reputable wildcrafters.

Tea: 1 1/2 to 3 teaspoons (3 to 6 grams) dried flower per cup, up to 3 ounces dried or 5 ounces fresh per quart, infused ten minutes. Take 1 cup three times a day.

Tincture: 1 teaspoon (5 milliliters) in water, three times a day, up to 6 ounces per week. Fresh plant glycerin: 1/2 to 1 teaspoon (2 1/2 to 5 milliliters), up to 4 ounces per week. Externally, a wash of the tea is used for burns, fungal infections of skin, and skin ulcers. External preparations may be used daily or frequently, whatever is practical.

ROSE, also called APOTHECARY'S ROSE. *Rosa gallica, R. canina, R. damascena.* **Parts used:** Flower, fruit (rosehips), essential oil. The essential oil from rose petals is used directly on skin, but because it takes sixty roses to make one drop of oil, the genuine product is expensive.

Indications: Rose petals or rosehips added in small amounts to tea mixtures imparts a delicate flavor; in addition, the scent released in an infusion has an effect through the olfactory nerves on the limbic region in the forebrain, associated with emotion, dream, and intuition. Rose is a symbol of love in every culture—every kind of love, including divine love and self-love.

Rose petals contain astringent tannins, making them a great addition to remedies for heavy bleeding at menses as well as spotting at menopause and in early pregnancy. They are also used for mild gastrointestinal infections accompanied by diarrhea and fever. Rosehips, which are high in vitamin C and bioflavonoids, improve iron absorption in anemic women or women experiencing heavy menstrual bleeding. Rosehips and rose petals are included in treatments for varicose veins to improve vessel tone. The antiseptic volatile oil and tannins in petals are also used externally in poultices to help heal a variety of skin eruptions, from eczema and psoriasis to acne, boils, and poorly healing wounds. In all uses, make sure you are using organically grown plants.

Tea: 1/2 to 1 teaspoon (1 to 2 grams) flowers or rosehips per cup, infused five minutes in a tightly covered container; 1 cup taken two to three times a day.

Tincture: 10 drops to 1 teaspoon (1 to 5 milliliters) in water, two to three times a day.

ROSEMARY. *Rosmarinus officinalis.* **Parts used:** Leaf, flowering top, essential oil.

Indications: Leaves and flowers are rich in aromatic oils that taste delicious and kill off unwanted microbes, especially in the digestive system but wherever tissue and herb have direct contact. Strewn in just-boiled water, the herb mingles its volatile oil with steam, which can be breathed in to clear congested sinuses and soothe headaches as well as upper respiratory inflammation. Used as an external wash for skin, the tea will correct a poor complexion. Used as a tea for internal cleansing, rosemary has a beneficial effect on blood circulation and elimination of excess fats. It improves circulation to the brain and has been known to improve memory and eyesight. A chemical in rosemary, diosmin, is thought to help reduce capillary fragility. Cosmetically, rosemary has been used for shampoo and hair rinses, especially for brunettes and redheads. Used daily from early adulthood on, it is said to postpone gray hair.

Contraindication: Rosemary is contraindicated during pregnancy in therapeutic doses given here. Occasional use in cooking and external aromatherapy is acceptable for most healthy women. If in doubt, avoid at this time.

Combinations: For its effect on capillary fragility and varicose veins, it combines well with horse chestnut *(Aesculus hippocastanum)*, yarrow *(Achillea millefolium)*, hawthorn *(Crataegus* species) and ginkgo *(Ginkgo biloba)*. However, it does take time, so be patient and, meanwhile, exercise as appropriate.

Tea: 1 teaspoon (2 grams) per cup, 1 ounce per pint up to 3 ounces per quart; take 1 cup two to four times daily.

Tincture: 1/3 to 1 teaspoon (15 drops to 5 milliliters), diluted in water, after eating, three times a day.

Essential oil: Two drops of the essential oil rubbed on the temples relieves a headache and in the bath reduces fatigue. Even a bath in rosemary tea is invigorating and replaces a twenty-minute catnap.

SAGE. *Salvia officinalis.* Red, black, and green sage are three varieties used. **Part used:** Leaf, gathered before or at the beginning of flowering in sunny weather, dried in the shade at low temperature.

Indications: Sage is known for its culinary flavor but has a wide variety of medicinal uses. This is not the same species as white sage, *Salvia apiana*, used in Native American ceremonies. A wild species, black sage, *S. mellifera,* shares many properties with *S. officinalis,* though it may be too medicinal tasting to use in cooking. The tea, especially of red sage, soothes a sore throat, including that of tonsillitis, and lowers fevers. Green sage, like all the sages, aids digestion, especially in counteracting heavy or fatty foods. Sage stimulates kidney excretion of bodily wastes, strengthens the lungs in asthma, calms the nerves in a mild way, and dries the milk of mothers who are weaning their babies, though in menopausal women it can improve skin, hair, and circulation with its hormonal tonic effects. It is useful for immune stresses at any age and is the classic remedy for inflammations of mucous membranes (sore throat, early sign of colds) and conditions of wet heat (for example, sweating). It is a local anti-inflammatory used for mouth ulcers, and a carminative, or gas-relieving remedy, for indigestion. It reduces diarrhea through a combination of its astringent, anti-inflammatory, and antiseptic effects.

Contraindication: Sage is too stimulating to uterine muscle contractions for use in medicinal amounts during pregnancy. Occasional culinary flavoring is usually fine for most women.

Combinations: Sage combines well with reproductive herbal remedies such as motherwort *(Leonurus cardiaca)*, raspberry leaf *(Rubus idaeus)*, and chasteberry *(Vitex agnus-castus)* for menopausal hot flashes. Sage also combines with licorice *(Glycyrrhiza glabra)* for sore throats and mixes well with chamomile *(Matricaria recutita)* for digestive disorders.

Tea: 1 to 2 teaspoons (2 to 4 grams) leaves steeped in 1 cup boiling water, covered, for ten minutes; use up to 1/2 to 1 ounce per pint, and take 1 cup three times a day.

Tincture: 1/2 to 2 teaspoons (2 1/2 to 10 milliliters) diluted in 1 cup water, herb tea, or juice, three times a day.

SARSAPARILLA, also called JAMAICAN SARSAPARILLA. *Smilax* species, *S. ornata*. **Part used:** Root.

Indications: Sarsaparilla is primarily used for improving nonspecific immunity; stimulating a rebalance of hormones; and cleansing itchy, scaly, or chronic skin conditions ranging from nervous hives to allergic reactions, psoriasis, and eczema. As a lymphatic tonic stimulating elimination, sarsaparilla has been used for clearing infections. In part because it contains anti-inflammatory phytosterols, sarsaparilla is perfectly suited to women with any range of problems affecting three inter-related "compartments" or body systems: immunity, lymph circulation, and skin. For this reason, it is part of a holistic treatment for women with systemic lupus erythematosus (SLE), rheumatoid arthritis, and other autoimmune conditions. Autoimmune conditions require attention beyond an herbal approach as these diseases are serious in nature.

Sarsaparilla has an effect on sex hormones and so is used to clear symptoms of premenstrual syndrome (PMS) and severe pain associated with the female reproductive system. It appears to help by reducing excess estrogen and affecting the nerves that sense pain, possibly via prostaglandin effects. Sarsaparilla is especially used for menopausal changes involving irregular cycles, mood swings, and skin problems (blemishes and dryness). Contrary to a common misconception, however, the root contains no testosterone. Its steroidal saponins are metabolized in such a way that they affect human hormonal balance, although the exact mechanism defies current testing methods and invites debate.

Sarsaparilla fell into disfavor with the orthodox medical establishment of Europe a few centuries ago, and its pharmacological mechanisms still have not been well researched, but its folk use as a reproductive tonic and a purifying herb for chronic disorders is well developed and precise. Native American women drank a tea of the root after delivery to expel the placenta. In China another species is used similarly to *S. ornata* in the West, as an alterative (cleansing tonic) for skin diseases, rheumatism, inflammation, and infections. Despite the herb's effects on hormonal balance, its promotion of elimination affects its own constituents, so that if the herb's hormonal sterols are not needed, they are readily excreted.

Caution: Taken in moderate dosage (see below) and starting only in the second trimester, the herb is considered a safe tonic for pregnant women with autoimmune or other chronic immune challenges. As always in pregnancy, begin with the lowest dose for one week before increasing to 2 grams decocted per cup, which may be taken for as long as three to five months depending on need, improvement in general health, the opinion of your health-care provider or midwife, and other considerations.

Combinations: For chronic conditions, sarsaparilla works well with immune-modulating herbs such as the Chinese herb huang chi *(Astragaulus membranaceus)*, *Echinacea* species, suma *(Pfaffia paniculata)*, and Siberian ginseng *(Eleutherococcus senticosus)*. Sarsaparilla is traditionally combined in "root beer," a compound tea, folk tincture, or fermented brew containing yellow dock root, dandelion root, burdock root, birch bark, and local herbal variations, including controversial sassafras bark in the southeastern United States. Root beer is used as a short-term cleansing tonic or to maintain health (1 to 2 cups tea or brew a day for two to three weeks each spring or autumn).

Tea: 1/2 to 1 1/2 teaspoons (1 to 3 grams) per cup, 1/2 ounce up to 1 ounce per pint, decocted fifteen minutes; 1 cup three times a day.

Tincture: 1/2 to 1 teaspoon (2 1/2 to 5 milliliters) in water, three times a day. Sarsaparilla extracts reasonably well as a glycerin tincture.

SHAVEGRASS. See HORSETAIL

SHEPHERD'S PURSE. *Capsella bursa-pastoris.* **Parts used:** Whole plant during seed stage. The dried herb has little use, especially if stored over four months.

Indications: Heavy menstrual bleeding with or without infection, fibroids, polyps, anemia caused by blood loss from the genito-urinary tract.

Shepherd's purse is the strongest of all astringents for promoting rapid blood clotting in any case of spotting, midcycle bleeding, flooding, or hemorrhage, and has been used successfully for uterine bleeding during emergencies in the absence of conventional medical care. Especially valuable because of its food-grade safety, it is a standard remedy for use during labor and delivery to slow or stop excess blood loss. In fact, it has been used as an ergot substitute for closing bleeding arteries of wounds and childbirth from the time of Hippocrates to World War I. It continues to be used by traditional midwives on four continents—the Americas, Europe, and Australia. In addition, because it is a member of the mustard family, it is safe taken over time for chronic internal bleeding problems, such as blood in urine or stool and uterine spotting, though all such conditions require diagnosis and attention. It is also a soothing diuretic for mild bladder infections. It is used externally as a wash for bleeding cuts and wounds. The fresh plant extract is diluted with water for a vaginal douche for discharges, inflammation of vaginal mucosa, and menopausal spotting. Discharges that do not respond in three days should be diagnosed before you decide to continue herbal self-help. Because it is a cooling and drying astringent, shepherd's purse is used for water retention caused by weak kidneys. It is also used for kidney stones, as it is said to be "favorable to the nephrons," the functional units of cells within the kidneys. It is used in France for treating varicose veins and hemorrhoids (distended blood vessels inside or at the rectum), taken orally as well as in hot sitz baths.

Whether you are taking an alcohol or glycerin extract or an infusion, use only fresh plant or the herb and seed dried within the last month. If you make fresh plant extract with alcohol, your preparation will taste and smell like yesterday's cooked Brussels sprouts, so to improve its palatability, add glycerin (10 percent by volume) to the tincture. You can also make an alcohol-free tincture with undiluted glycerin and fresh plant.

Caution: People with sensitive skin may experience irritation from handling the fresh shepherd's purse, which contains mustard oils. However, the fresh plant extract or tea give no similar reaction, even when taken by sensitive people.

Combinations: Shepherd's purse combines well with yarrow for cystitis, especially interstitial cystitis.

Tea: 1/2 to 1 ounce fresh plant per 8-ounce cup; a strong infusion of 3 to 4 ounces per quart, 1 cup every hour as needed or three times a day, works internally and also as a douche.

Tincture: 10 drops to 2 teaspoons (1 to 10 milliliters), repeated as needed every twenty minutes or three times a day, usually up to 2 ounces per week, or 2 ounces per day in extreme need and under supervision of a qualified health-care professional.

SIBERIAN GINSENG. *Eleutherococcus senticosus.* **Part used:** Root.

Indications: Siberian ginseng is an *adaptogen,* a tonic that is harmless, has nonspecific effects (that is, it is effective for a wide variety of conditions), and normalizes the body toward health. For example, if the body is overstimulated, Siberian ginseng is relaxing but never *too* relaxing. If the body is too sluggish or weakened, it is energizing, but unlike its stronger cousin, ginseng *(Panax ginseng)*, it is rarely overstimulating; nor does it cause headaches or other symptoms associated with overuse; and it is more affordable for long-term use.

Conditions for which Siberian ginseng is given include chronic reproductive infections, hormonal imbalance linked to emotional stress, arthritis, high blood pressure, hardened arteries and heart disease, high or low blood sugar, lung conditions such as emphysema or chronic bronchitis, damage from trauma and even cancer. Siberian ginseng is used to balance out the hormones during periods of intense physical change, including the postpartum and any stage of the Change from peri- to postmenopause. It is particularly useful when stress worsens a woman's main health complaint. It is also given to those with weak systems that need a thorough overhaul without stimulation. Though the root increases energy reserves and stamina, it does so by nourishing the body's natural mechanisms.

Siberian ginseng can be used long term to assist in altering long-standing stress and thereby make long-lasting improvements to immunity, mental clarity, and mood. In traditional Asian and eastern Russian use, the root is given to promote a long life with vigorous energy. It is also given to improve memory and to get the best-quality work from someone under stressful conditions that cannot be altered. It is commonly taken by athletes to improve physical performance and endurance. For the latter reason it is also given to those who must maintain both clarity of mind and physical well-being in the midst of extreme emotional intensity, such as mountain rescue teams.

Siberian ginseng has been studied extensively in large groups of humans since the early 1960s under a number of circumstances, including normal working conditions. Normal work in this case means anything from high-stress management to repetitive factory jobs to simply too much work and not enough joy. Though the best effects happen over time, two to three days of moderate-to-high dosage will bring short-term benefits to immunity, mental function, and stress response, including stabilized blood sugar levels. Stability despite heat, noise, exercise, increased workload, and mental stress may well prove the effectiveness of Siberian ginseng. Furthermore, there is no dropoff in efficiency and general good mood when the herb has had enough time to work its magic and is eventually discontinued. It is best taken for a minimum of two months, after which women can skip one day per week or one week every six weeks. This is not because of toxic accumulation but rather because the lower dose will help stimulate the body to slowly recover its own natural means for adapting to stress.

Note: If regular use has little to no effect in one to two months, the herb may be wrongly labeled. Two common substitutes in the herb trade are *E. gracilistylus* (unproven; may be similar or weaker) or Indian sarsaparilla *(Hemidesmus indica, H. periploca)*, which has other uses but none of the properties of Siberian ginseng. Buy from reputable herb dealers or politely, insistently request a better grade at your local herb store.

Caution: Some women still having regular menstrual cycles have reported that Siberian ginseng increased breast tenderness at normal doses; this seems to indicate that it is not the right herbal adaptogen for them no matter what their stress level may be. This side effect has not been reported by menopausal or postmenopausal women.

Tea: 1/2 to 2 1/2 teaspoons (1 to 5 grams) decocted per cup, 1/2 to 2 ounces per pint, 1 cup one to four times a day. Water extract (tea) of good-quality herb works well and may even have more of the beneficial polysaccharides than tincture.

Tincture: For sensitive or very ill people, effective doses may be as little as 5 drops. For stronger effects, use 1 teaspoon (5 milliliters) once a day. For chronic conditions in strong individuals, a moderate dose is 1/2 teaspoon (2 1/2 milliliters), but there is a safe range upward to 1/2 ounce (15 milliliters) tincture, this dose taken one to three times a day. In these higher doses, teas, tablets, capsules, and glycerin extracts may be preferred to alcohol tinctures because of the price and volume of extract consumed. Homemade extracts work well, and Siberian ginseng powder extracts moderately well in glycerin and water (see "Herbal Preparations" later in this book).

SKULLCAP. *Scutellaria lateriflora, S. galericulata.* **Parts used:** Leaf, gathered in early flowering stages; even store-bought dried herb should yield some tiny dried blue flower pieces on close examination. The root of a different species, *S. baicalensis,* is used in traditional Chinese medicine as a digestive tonic for improving liver function. These two kinds of skullcap are not interchangeable.

Indications: This herb is highly regarded among herbalists for nervous tension, premenstrual syndrome (PMS), and insomnia. As a relaxing nervine tea, skullcap can be mixed with many other herbs or combinations. Its taste is pleasant but bland, not minty.

Skullcap is given for those with long stretches of PMS or women in menopause with severe mood changes every month. It takes at least three consecutive months of a skullcap combination to shift the hormones permanently. It does restore some function in exhausted nervous people, so it is given to those with poor memory or concentration when these symptoms are combined with insomnia or chronic fatigue. It tends to promote sleep when taken for that purpose but is not as strong a sedative as hops or valerian. When these two herbs are too heavy for sensitive people, skullcap is preferred. In low-to-moderate doses, skullcap can be given during the day without the side effect of drowsiness. Preliminary research suggests it may have antiallergic action.

Tea: 1 to 2 teaspoons (2 to 4 grams) per cup, up to 1 ounce per pint, infused, 1 cup three times a day. For help in getting to sleep, use 1 1/2 ounces per pint; drink half (3 to 4 ounces) an hour before bedtime and the other half in bed. If nighttime urination is a concern, drink smaller amounts, void bladder before bedtime, or use the more concentrated tincture. For extreme agitation or pain, including that of PMS and cramps, tincture is more effective than tea.

Tincture: 1/2 to 1 teaspoon (2 1/2 to 5 milliliters) diluted in a little water, one to four times a day; use a maximum of 4 ounces per week. In the short term, take tincture, 1 teaspoon (5 milliliters), every ten to twenty minutes as needed, up to 12 doses spread over the day and night, or 2 ounces (60 milliliters) in twenty-four hours.

STINGING NETTLE. See NETTLE

ST. JOHN'S WORT. *Hypericum perforatum.* **Part used:** Flowering top, harvested at the peak of flowering before noon on dry days, traditionally St. John's Day, June 21, which is also the summer solstice. The dried flowering tops can be used for oil, tea, or tincture, but the fresh plant extracts are stronger.

Some women in the Wiccan or pagan tradition call St. John's wort "St. Joan's wort" after Joan of Arc to signify its many strengthening aspects.

Indications: St. John's wort is given for all inflamed conditions of the nerves, including viral infections such as herpes. Modern German and Russian clinical research shows it kills several bacteria. It is an anti-inflammatory for internal or external swellings, inflammations, and bleeding wounds. It helps the body repair, and it promotes growth of granulation tissue for minimal scarring after severe burns.

The newest findings show its efficacy in preventing infection in immune-compromised people, such as those on conventional cancer therapy, and HIV-positive people.

The red flower oil is used externally on painful shingles eruptions, often in combination with nerve-numbing menthol or peppermint essential oil and/or garlic oil. As a nerve pain remedy, it is given externally and internally for sciatica or nerve endings damaged by trauma. As a tissue restorative for nerves and skin, St. John's wort is indicated for stroke patients, sleepwalkers, and accident victims, as well as for people with mild neuroses. It is a specific tonic for debilitated nerves and is given for melancholy and exhaustion. Used as an antidepressant, it takes six to eight weeks for its beneficial effects to be felt. To lessen anxiety and mood swings, it may take a few doses or a few days, depending on severity. Chemicals in the herb, hypericins, have a monoamine oxidase–inhibiting mode of action, which means the herb should not be used with other antidepressant drugs that are monoamine oxidase inhibiting without informing your health-care provider.

St. John's wort has a paraxodical effect that makes it a great tonic during menopause: it moistens dry tissues while drying up excess discharges or bleeding, including spotting between cycles. Because it reduces bleeding, it is also given for problems as different as blood from severe coughing; hard growths, especially breast cancer; varicose veins; and humble but irritating hemorrhoids (distended blood vessels in or near rectum).

Contraindications: In sensitive people, the hypericin in St. John's wort can cause a light sensitivity of eyes and skin that usually disappears within three or four days after stopping use. The main reports come from use of extraconcentrated products or direct handling of the fresh cut plant in flower. When St. John's wort is used for three consecutive months or longer, which is the best way to get the full complement of antidepressant and preventative immune and neurological effects, avoiding full-summer sun is advisable. These problems do not occur as often with the normal doses listed below or in external use of the plant as a poultice on open, infected wounds or as an ointment on irritated, dry skin.

Tea: 1 to 2 teaspoons (2 to 4 grams) per cup, 1 ounce per pint, infused; 1 cup three times a day.

Tincture: 10 drops to 1 teaspoon (1 to 5 milliliters) diluted in water, three times a day.

External oil: To prepare, fill a jar with fresh flowers and buds only (few to no leaves); then cover with a light, cold-pressed vegetable oil such as safflower, almond, or odorless sesame. Keep the jar at a warm temperature for ten days; then strain the oil. Use it directly on bruises, wounds, and burns, or incorporate it into salves and ointments. See "Herbal Preparations" later in this book.

SUMA, also called PARA TODO. *Pfaffia paniculata.* **Part used:** Root. The dried root comes in chips or as powder; it tastes like peanuts but is slightly bitter. The leaves are used in herbal beverage tea but do not have the same strength of the root.

Indications: Suma has four main areas of medicinal use: (1) reproductive, including conditions such as infertility, premenstrual syndrome (PMS), menopausal hot flashes, vaginal atrophy, and insomnia linked with mood swings; (2) immunity, including chronic degenerative diseases such as cancer, autoimmune disease, and AIDS, probably because it contains germanium, pfaffic acids, and pfaffosides; (3) endocrine balance for abnormalities of blood sugar metabolism, including both hypoglycemia and diabetes, because it contains germanium and polysaccharides; (4) wound healing and restorative properties, probably because it contains allantoin and germanium. Though medical and pharmacological universities from South America through Europe to Japan have tested it, analysis raises more questions than it answers because some constituents are new to science and the whole-plant extract works better than each individual component. For at least three hundred years the root has been used as a tonic food for the elderly or debilitated and a rejuvenating source of energy, as well as to treat malignant tumors and diabetes. It became known as Brazilian ginseng (though it is not related). Brazilian hospitals and Japanese pharmaceutical companies have research to support suma's traditional use in providing multiple health benefits. In Europe, South America, and Japan, suma has been used in cancer clinics for shrinking tumors and rebuilding tissue health, especially after standard cancer therapies. Suma is given internally for Hodgkins, leukemia, lymphoma, stomach, bowel, skin, and breast cancer. It is being given on an experimental basis to HIV-positive and AIDS patients, with preliminary results showing promise for long-term survival so far, yet its immume benefits are still only cause for cautious optimism. As a possible treatment for diabetes, it has been shown at the University of São Paulo, Brazil, to restimulate the insulin-producing cells of the pancreas in instances where some functional capability has been present, but long-term studies have yet to be translated and made widely available for review. At the least, suma seems to synergize with insulin, thereby allowing non-insulin-dependent diabetics to control blood sugar through diet and possibly allowing others to gradually use lower insulin doses, thereby lowering long-term side effects of the injections and disease.

As a wound healer, suma is applied externally to open or poorly healing wounds. Its vitamin C content may combine with other factors for regeneration of epithelial cell layers. It does not have the same caution as allantoin-containing comfrey *(Symphytum officinale)*, as suma does not stimulate superficial skin repair faster than the layers below. Whether or not suma is an adaptogen in the strict sense that ginseng and Siberian ginseng are, it is clear that the root has an ability to help people adapt to stress.

Suma is given to those who are trying to lose weight, as it stimulates metabolism while lowering excess blood sugar and lessening craving for refined sweets. People report that after a few weeks they sleep a little less but wake up a little more refreshed, without the alarm clock or the need for coffee. It seems to "rev" up the engine without a midafternoon crash, so it can be given when endurance is required.

Contraindications: Because it is a stimulant of reproductive hormones, suma is unsafe in the first trimester of pregnancy. However, in Brazil, where malnutrition is epidemic, suma is given as a tonic food in doses under 3 grams a day, beginning in the second trimester, to women who may not maintain health throughout pregnancy, with no side effects reported in mothers or children after delivery.

Notes on preparation: Suma can be taken as tea, tincture, capsules, or powder. The best way to take powder in the higher range of doses may be in starch paper or as a gruel, 1 to 2 teaspoons per cup of water. To make the mixture more palatable, add a teaspoon of honey or natural sweetener (except in cases of diabetes or blood sugar problems), vanilla or almond extract, or a drop of peppermint oil per 8-ounce cup of water. This starchy gruel may also be combined in a fresh fruit smoothie or similar healthy blender drink. In reproductive conditions excluding first-trimester pregnancy, you can take suma in 4-to-5-gram doses, prepared as above. For effective results in regulating blood sugar, a gradual increase up to 8 to 10 grams a day has been found necessary, but this regimen requires careful monitoring in diabetics.

Tea: 1/2 to 1 1/2 teaspoons (1 to 3 grams) per cup, up to 1 ounce per pint, infused (though a root because powdered herb allows extraction) for twenty minutes; take 1 cup one to three times a day.

Tincture: 1/2 to 1 teaspoon (2 1/2 to 5 milliliters) diluted in water, three to six times a day.

TANG KWEI. See DONG QUAI

UVA-URSI. See BEARBERRY

VALERIAN. *Valeriana officinalis.* **Parts used:** Root, rootlet. Good-quality dried root pieces are yellow-brown with brittle rootlets and have a bitter taste that is both pungent and camphorlike. Older dried root smells and tastes like old socks, but it still works.

Indications: The dried roots make a pungent herb tea or extract used to prevent or break the cycle of insomnia or to take the edge off pain. Valerian is the ideal tranquilizer, not a true sedative, as it does not truly reduce sensitivity or motor control. When taken by someone experiencing both exhaustion and agitation, it acts as a sedative. It can reduce reflex nervous response and activity in the psychomotor sphere (when you've had too much to think). In cases of extreme fatigue, valerian acts as an equalizing nervine remedy. Because the volatile components of the herb act on nerves as well as relaxing muscles, it is given to relieve menstrual or ovulation cramps, to relax jittery muscles, and to settle mood swings. It is especially indicated when these problems bring disturbed sleep, which in turn worsens hormonal changes, especially in menopause. Older people in particular report that they use valerian to get to sleep more quickly and that it does not affect dream recall. Valerian has also been used with good effect for settling gastrointestinal pain accompanied by bloating and spasms of colic.

Valerian is a woman's herb, and not just to keep her quiet and happy. It buys time while a woman regathers her energies. The root is strongly relaxing when the physical body and mental/emotional being are out of sync with each other, as when, for example, a woman is burning the candle at both ends to get a series of near-impossible chores done, dealing with a typically destructive modern workweek while her body is going through menopause, or taking care of an older parent without adequate backup support. Valerian brings release from muscle tension and nervous tension. It may be given to fragile women and those with a fragile nervous system.

Valerian root can be used in moderation for a bad spell of high stress when a vacation is not possible. Though it is not a tonic—it cannot be taken long term in large amounts—leaning into *Valeriana*'s rooty arms brings special strength. The sleep-producing and pain-relieving effects are temporary and not habit forming, unlike the prescription sedative drug Valium, which is a benzodiazepine. Valium acts differently in our bodies and is not chemically related in any way to valerian.

Contraindications: Normally, valerian doesn't interact with other common prescription drugs or even barbiturates, but people on antipsychotic or other mood-altering drugs may be oversensitive to the plant and could have unexpected and undesirable reactions. Because alcohol does interact negatively with barbiturates, replace sleeping pills with moderate doses of the tincture (don't combine) or use a nonalcohol form of the herb (capsules, glycerites).

Every once in a while a person is reported to have a paradoxical reaction with valerian, becoming headachey and anxious at low to moderate dosage. If this happens to you, switch to passion flower or skullcap. Common-sense use of valerian for short-term insomnia, pain, or tension during pregnancy is safe.

Cautions: The biochemicals in valerian, valepotriates, were once considered by some as possibly unsafe, but only because tests were performed on isolated chemicals injected into lab animals rather than herb preparations taken orally. Toxicity tests have shown valerian to be remarkably safe compared to tranquilizers and muscle-relaxing drugs. Excess amounts probably act on the central nervous system as a depressant (like excess alcohol).

Be aware that if you need valerian to turn off the tension so a good night's sleep can prepare you for another busy day, more is not better. Instead, start with standard doses earlier in the evening and plan for a stretch of deep sleep. If your body is bone tired, valerian will screen out everything except your body's need for sleep, including that buzzing alarm clock. If you are sensitive to medication, begin with low doses and increase within the ranges given until it works.

Clinical trials found that a hangover effect or headache was difficult to get with valerian, though consumers reported that it was a concern. You cannot easily take too much unless you take concentrated alcohol tinctures without waiting ten to twenty minutes for each dose to take effect. An excess causes irritability and headaches, with a dull, morning stupor. The root's distinctive stinkiness may disagree with some people, though it may be one way Nature keeps us from using her tranquilizing nerve medicine too often!

Combinations: Valerian combines well with hops *(Humulus lupulus)*, especially when tension, pain, or worry (treated by valerian) is accompanied by agitation or overexcitation (treated by hops). This combination has a pretty bad taste, however, so you will likely prefer tincture or glycerites to cups of tea; capsules take a while to have effect. A classic triad for insomnia is equal parts of valerian, hops, and passion flower *(Passiflora incarnata)*. Valerian also combines well with lemon balm *(Melissa officinalis)* for a milder calming effect during the day.

Note on preparation: Even though this is a root, valerian contains volatile oils and so must be infused or steeped (not decocted or boiled). Steep fifteen to twenty minutes, well covered. Fresh root tea and tincture are stronger than dried herb preparations.

Tea: The range is large, from 1/4 to 2 1/2 teaspoons (1/2 to 5 grams), 1/4 ounce up to 2 ounces per 3 cups; take 1 to 3 cups at a time as needed. Most adults who need valerian can take 100-milligram tablets or capsules with water three times a day without experiencing daytime drowsiness. Taking capsules or tablets up to 500 milligrams per dose at night can help the most stubborn insomnia, though relief may not occur until after several nights at this dose.

Tincture: 10 drops to 1 teaspoon (1 to 5 milliliters) three times a day or more often. If you are in acute pain or nervous states, repeat every fifteen minutes. You can take extra doses or a couple of large doses at night for sleep or for pain, up to 2 ounces tincture diluted in water (or strong, hot valerian tea) at a time. Pain thresholds differ markedly among people, so that one woman may do well with a few drops while another needs a big gulp. Experiment within these ranges to find the dose for your best response to this worthy herbal tranquilizer.

VERBENA. See VERVAIN

VERVAIN, also called BLUE VERVAIN or VERBENA. *Verbena officinalis.* **Parts used:** Leaf, stem, collected before or during midflowering.

Indications: Vervain is a stimulating physical tonic after prolonged illness, but it is a relaxing remedy as well. It has been used for everything from bringing down fevers to promoting healthy breast milk in tense young mothers to stimulating the rebalancing of female sex hormones, possibly through combined effects on the liver's breakdown of hormones and endocrine gland functions. It has a weak parasympathomimetic activity and no-to-low toxicity. As a liver and digestive tonic, vervain helps clear chronic toxic conditions, including congestion of the spleen. It helps prevent the formation of some gallstones by changing the consistency of bile, stimulating its earlier release before it is fully concentrated in the gallbladder, by generally increasing the moisture in the digestive system, and by relaxing any tightness of muscles in the bile ducts. It is also used in German and Dutch traditions for kidney stones. As a bitter stimulant to digestive metabolism, vervain may bring on a menstrual cycle, especially one blocked with constipation or pelvic sluggishness. Its traditional folkloric use is to cleanse away "obstructions that need opening."

As a nervine, vervain is a mild relaxant but a strong tonic. It is given over a period of one to three months for stubborn depression with physical signs of depressed immunity. Large doses used in the short term for immediate effects seem to work better than small ones for nervous exhaustion. Vervain is often given in small amounts (it is quite bitter) to sweeten a critical, fussy nature or to soften those whose attitudes are "hard."

Used externally, as a wound-healing herb, vervain astringes or reduces bleeding, disinfects, and is considered to bring the maternal kiss of Nature to the blows encountered in life. The powdered herb is widely used for treating infected gums, tooth decay, bad breath, sore throats, and dry mouth.

Contraindications: Vervain's bitter effect is stimulating to digestion and peristalsis, so it may worsen active ulcers. It is unsafe in early pregnancy or where there is danger of increased peristalis causing a miscarriage.

Combinations: Though unrelated botanically, lemon verbena and vervain make a great pair, the sweet citrus aroma mellowing the bitter kick of the other. Vervain is specific for migraine caused by anxiety and tension or menstrual imbalance, as opposed to food allergies; for that purpose it combines well with fresh feverfew extract *(Chrysanthemum parthenium)* or wood betony *(Stachys betonica)*. In depression associated with a locked-up quality (heavy tension, high blood pressure, irritable bowel syndrome), vervain combines well with either cramp bark or black haw *(Viburnum* species).

Tea: 1 to 2 teaspoons (2 to 4 grams) per cup, 1 to 2 ounces per pint; take 1 cup three times a day before meals.

Tincture: 1 teaspoon (5 milliliters) in water, three times a day. Because it has a bitter flavor and its alkaloids extract reasonably well in glycerin, vervain makes a fine glycerin tincture, especially with fresh leaf.

WILD OATS, also called OATSTRAW. *Avena sativa.* **Parts used:** The fresh green plant: stem, leaf, but especially seed.

Indications: Nervous exhaustion, frazzled nerve endings, insomnia, tension headaches, poor tolerance to pain, adrenal weakness, chronic constipation, and malnutrition. Its high mineral content make it an ideal long-term tonic for bones, hair, and nails. Oats are an excellent restorative in almost all cases of deficiency. The herb is given in the context of whole-person support to offset substance abuse or ease the transition. Oats can also help those who are living "clean" yet feel as if they aren't. It may help antiviral herbs (St. John's wort, lemon balm) reduce herpes outbreaks.

Contraindication: Contraindicated in Celiac's disease, an autoimmune digestive condition characterized by a missing enzyme and the resulting intolerance to gluten.

Special preparation: Fresh plant tincture (1:2 weight-to-volume ratio) is most effective. Fresh seed juice may be preserved with glycerin or as alcohol extracts.

Tea: 1/2 to 1 1/2 teaspoons (1 to 3 grams) per cup, 1/2 to 1 ounce per pint, standard infusion; take 1 cup tea one to three times a day. Can be taken indefinitely.

Tincture: 1/4 to 1 teaspoon three times a day, up to six times a day for extreme agitation or insomnia. Children and sensitive people should begin at the lower dose and gradually increase as needed. The standard adult dose of tincture ranges from 1/2 teaspoon up to a maximum of 3 ounces per day, but the higher doses must have reasonable justification (severe pain, acute loss, grieving) and then may only be continued for one to two weeks before professional supervision is indicated.

WILD YAM. *Dioscorea villosa.* **Part used:** Root. This is one of the hardest herbs to grind once it is dry and has broken many a kitchen coffee grinder and blender. In commerce it comes as odorless yellow-brown chips or powder. It tastes bland at first, then turns acrid.

Indications: Wild yam is given for reproductive spasm, pain, and inflammation. It is classically given for uterine pain, such as severe menstrual pain, or shooting pain beyond cramps. Wild yam is also used for ovarian spasm and inflammation, such as occurs with pelvic inflammatory disease (PID) or painful ovulation. The root has the same healing effects in the digestive system and so is a specific tonic for painful spasm with inflammation, such as that occasioned by diverticulitis. It is useful as part of a natural approach to any endocrine imbalance. Its steroidal saponins are the basis for the birth control pill and other anti-inflammatories. For this reason it is sometimes expensive, because pharmaceutical firms buy up large crops on the global market. The side effects of steroidal drugs are thankfully absent from use of this herb. Wild yam, given in combination with black cohosh *(Cimicifuga racemosa)*, is not only common in menopause formulas but is also an effective pain-relieving remedy for rheumatoid arthritis, especially in the inflamed stages of flare-up.

Note: Powder in capsules is observed to give a minor side effect of intestinal gas.

Tea: 1 to 2 teaspoons (2 to 4 grams) per cup, 1/2 to 2 ounces per pint or 3 cups; take 1 cup three times a day.

Tincture: 1 teaspoon (5 milliliters) three times a day.

WILLOW. *Salix alba.* **Part used:** Bark.

Indications: Willow is used for arthritic joint pain, aching muscles, and general malaise (feeling of being unwell or "under the weather"). It is not irritating to sensitive digestive tracts so can be taken easily where other anti-inflammatories may not be well tolerated. It reduces fevers and is indicated when infection aggravates bone or joint disease.

Tea: 1 to 2 teaspoons (2 to 4 grams) per cup, up to 3 ounces per pint decocted; take 1/2 cup three times a day.

Tincture: 1 to 3 teaspoons (5 to 15 milliliters) diluted in water, one to six times a day as needed.

YAM. See WILD YAM

YARROW. *Achillea millefolium.* **Parts used:** Leaf and flower.

Indications: Used internally, this universal remedy optimizes six body systems: the cardiovascular, respiratory, immune, urinary, digestive, and reproductive systems. It is given for heavy bleeding; its astringency combines with its stimulating effects on the liver to assist in balancing hormones while helping the body shrink fibroids. It is used for sluggish metabolism combined with irregular cycles with or without spotting and flooding around menopause. Yarrow is cooling as a cold tea or tincture, useful for hot flashes and night sweats. Hot drinks of yarrow bring on perspiration and may be used for cleansing or bringing down fevers. When high blood pressure, sensitivity to heat, and indigestion occur in combination before or after menopause, yarrow is indicated. The young leaves taste bitter but are nutritious. A simple tea can be used as a wash for infected cuts and wounds.

Contraindications: Yarrow is contraindicated in pregnancy and with photosensitivity (sensitivity to light).

Combinations: Combined with hawthorn and linden, it brings down high blood pressure; used with elder and peppermint, it is a classic tea for reducing fevers.

Tea: 1 to 2 teaspoons (2 to 4 grams) infused per cup, up to 1/2 ounce dried herb per pint or 1 ounce per quart. Take 1/2 cup or more as desired three times a day.

Tincture: 1/2 to 1 teaspoon diluted in a cup of water, three times a day, with a normal limit of 2 1/2 ounces of extract per week.

YELLOW DOCK, also called CURLY DOCK. *Rumex crispus.* **Part used:** Root. Harvest roots when the plant is at least 2 1/2 feet high and after seeds have dropped. The older the plant, the larger the root.

Indications: Yellow dock root is given to people with chronic skin conditions and is especially used by those with congestive dysmenorrhea. Conditions it can help include menstrual cramps with a tendency toward constipation, acne outbreaks, and cystic or seborrheic blemishes. It is given for any skin eruption to speed the body's complete removal of inflammatory conditions and is especially terrific for itching conditions. Yellow dock is a stimulating but mild laxative used for chronic bloating, gas, and indigestion. It can be given in mild or severe constipation, short term or long.

Students of phytopharmacology may be interested to note that the oxalate-containing yellow dock root has been given with great results to people with sour stomach, even though an excess of oxalic acid on its own is a powerful poison that destroys the structure of tissues, especially in the digestive tract. In the case of diarrhea or alternating constipation and diarrhea with irritable bowel syndrome, the stimulating laxative effects of yellow dock are less irritating than stronger herbal laxatives because of its action on the liver and the gallbladder's secretion of bile, which is the body's own natural laxative. The herb does promote elimination of metabolic toxins through the bowel, helpful when the other organs of elimination (skin, lungs, kidney) are overstressed. This may be indicated by eczema, psoriasis, other chronic skin problems, rashes, allergy, and hayfever, (all of which may get worse at menses), chronic bronchitis, and chronic bladder infections.

Since it promotes the flow of bile, which metabolizes dietary fats for elimination, yellow dock is used to bring down cholesterol and clean the system. The root is rich in minerals, including a nonconstipating blend of iron and other essential nutrients, for those with chronic fatigue, poor blood quality, or anemia. If anemia is due to excess bleeding, the toning effect that yellow dock has on the liver makes it a useful addition to herbal combinations aimed at hepatic rebalancing of the hormones.

Yellow dock contains significant amounts of vitamin C, which assists in assimilation when one is taking iron, though percentages vary from source to source.

Yellow dock's astringent and purifying effect is said to promote healthy blood flow to the sweat and digestive glands, partially explaining its alterative, tonic effect. Yellow dock works on chronic skin conditions in the long term, for at least three consecutive months before lasting change may be seen. Yellow dock is much milder and more strengthening than the harsher cathartic or laxative herbs that also contain anthraquinones. Examples of those include senna (*Cassia* species), *Cascara sagrada (Rhamnus purshiana)*, and purging buckthorn *(R. cathartica)*.

Caution: Yellow dock is not as bad as herbal anthraquinone laxatives (senna and the others) in pregnancy or sensitive women, but caution is wise. If bowel pain occurs, drink large amounts (8 to 24 ounces) of hot water, fennel tea, and/or other carminative herbs to reduce painful peristalsis (movement) and spasm of the intestines. If symptoms haven't improved within two hours, you're better safe than sorry—call your health-care provider.

Note: Other than in pregnancy, yellow dock is considered a safe herb when taken in doses listed below.

Combinations: Yellow dock combines well with burdock *(Arctium lappa)* for its cleansing effects on skin and the blood or for chronic degenerative diseases, including arthritis. For heavy menstrual bleeding, it combines well with shepherd's purse *(Capsella bursa-pastoris)* or yarrow *(Achillea millefolium)*. An externally applied poultice of crushed green leaves (highest in vitamin C) is used to treat allergic or nervous hives, ringworm, and other fungal infections of the skin. Roots extracted in vinegar may also be used on ringworm.

Tea: 1 to 2 teaspoons (2 to 4 grams) decocted per cup, up to 1 ounce per pint; take 1 tablespoon to 1 cup of tea three times a day.

Tincture: 1/2 teaspoon as needed, usually 1 1/2 teaspoons per day, up to 1 2/3 ounces per week. Best taken before meals for sluggish absorption of nutrients or before bed for constipation (works overnight for A.M. release in one to four days).

Appendix A

Guidelines for Preparing Herbs

Extracts

Also called "tinctures" (TINK-shures), these concentrated herbal preparations last indefinitely, unlike teas, and can be taken in small amounts. Five to 10 drops of tincture diluted in a little water may be the most effective way to take a remedy, not to mention more convenient than brewing up a pot of tea. Some women find that 3 teaspoons of tincture, diluted in a little juice, herb tea, or water, sipped over ten minutes, does the trick in twenty minutes, whereas a tea may take longer—twenty minutes to an hour.

Not all active chemical constituents in herbs are water soluble, so alcohol or another solvent is usually necessary to fully extract the herb's properties. Vegetable glycerin (GLIH-sa-rin) is a commonly used solvent; even vinegar can be an effective solvent for some herbs. Tinctures in alcohol bases are the most commonly available commercially, and the amount of alcohol per dose is relatively small. If, however, you are unable to use alcohol-based herb preparations, you can readily replace them with glycerin- or other nonalcohol-based extracts, herb teas, aromatherapy, and even herb oils for absorption through the skin. A common belief is that adding boiling water to alcohol tinctures burns off the alcohol, and this helps, but some alcohol is left afterward and some heat-sensitive herb properties may be lost.

Dosage varies depending on whether an extract contains one herb or a combination, the herbs themelves, and who it is taking it. A general guideline is to use 1/2 to 1 teaspoon in 1/2 to 1 cup of water three times a day. Small or sensitive women may start with 1/2 teaspoon; those with strong constitutions or more demanding health concerns find that a beginning dose of 1 teaspoon to be more effective. Glycerin tinctures are usually less potent than alcohol tinctures, so you can take a little more.

Tinctures are expensive in retail herb shops and health-food stores, so you may want to make your own. They are easy to make, and in the doses recommended in this book they are far more effective and affordable than retail products. Whether you are using one herb or a combination, place 5 ounces in a blender or food processor and shred the material into small pieces (but it needn't be a powder);

then put it into a glass jar or other container with a tight lid. Add 25 ounces of at least 40 percent alcohol (80 proof or stronger, such as medium-priced brandy or vodka). Shake the closed container to evenly mix liquid and herb pieces, once every day for fourteen days. Store out of direct light and away from heat sources (a convenient spot in your kitchen cupboard, for instance). After two weeks, strain the mixture through a piece of clean muslin large enough that you can wrap it up and squeeze out the last few drops of liquid. Store the extract in a dark glass bottle with a lid (a brown bottle from your drugstore or a sterilized green wine bottle with a cork). Label the container with the date, name of herb, name of person it is for, and the dose.

Tinctures do not require refrigeration; store capped tightly away from direct heat, light, and children.

Teas

Herbal teas can be steeped (infused) or simmered (decocted).

Infusions

Leaves, flowers, and delicate parts of plants with fragrance are best steeped, 1 ounce of dried herb to three 8-ounce cups of just-boiled water. Put the herb in a teapot or nonmetal container, pour the water over the herb, and cover with a well-fitting lid. Allow the tea to sit, or steep, for five to twenty-five minutes, usually about fifteen, before straining out the herb and discarding it. Drink from 1/2 to 1 cup of tea two to three times a day. In the "Tea" information given in the "Materia Medica" section in this book, 1 teaspoon is said to be equivalent to 2 grams, but this is inexact because of variation in herb density; therefore, the section also provides weights, such as 1 ounce to a pint.

Decoctions

The tough parts of herbs, such as roots, bark, seeds, and berries, are placed in cold water, 1 ounce of dried herb to 3 cups of water, in a stainless steel or other suitable vessel covered with a well-fitting lid. Bring the pot to a simmer over low heat and leave it at the lowest possible heat for five to twenty-five minutes, usually fifteen, before straining out the herb and discarding it. Take 1/2 to 1 cup of tea two to three times a day.

Many herb combinations contain both leaves and flowers as well as roots and seeds. If you have the time, you can separately simmer the roots, bark, berries, and seeds in the total amount of water and for the time period called for; then turn off the heat and add the leaves, flowers, and herbs, and let them steep for the usual fifteen minutes or the specified time before straining. Seeds or other materials that have a strong aroma because they contain volatile oils should be added at the steeping step. This method results in the strongest combinations. If you are short on time, the combinations in this book will work just fine if you prepare the herbs all at once; just let the roots and leaves sit, or steep, an extra few minutes. Combinations using extracts do not require any special preparation: each root or flower has already been extracted so you just combine them and take as directed.

Sweeten teas with a little honey if you wish, but do not use refined sugar. You can make enough tea to last three days, store it in the refrigerator, and drink it hot or cold or at room temperature; you can also reheat a cup at a time. Herb tea will not last longer than three days, even covered and refrigerated.

How long should you take these teas? No book can pretend to know exactly in each woman's case, but as a guide, acute problems should respond in a few doses or a few days. These are best treated with a dose every ten to twenty minutes or at least every one to two hours as needed until you feel better. Then take one dose two to three times a day for another few days. In cases of infection, continue taking herbs for seven to ten days past the acute stage to help the body's recovery and prevent recurrence.

Chronic conditions should show some sign of improvement in one to three weeks even if all symptoms do not respond at once. For the best outcome, take herbs three times a day for at least one to three months, in some cases up to a year for permanent improvement.

External Preparations: Herbal Oils and Salves

Many herbs, such as wild yam, comfrey, calendula, and St. John's wort, can be extracted in oil and then applied externally or vaginally daily and during intercourse for lubrication. Or you can add essential oils like lavender, clary sage, and jasmine to them and use them as massage and bath oils.

To make an herbal oil, place 4 ounces of dried herb in a clean, dry quart jar, shake the herbs to settle them, and add green unfiltered olive oil, sesame oil, or almond oil to 1 inch above the level of herb in the container. Cover with a well-fitting but not completely tightened lid, place the jar in a saucepan of water, and keep on low heat for three days. Or, if you will not be at home, leave the jar in a constantly warm place (top of refrigerator or water heater) or in the sun for ten days.

At the end of this time, strain out the herb material and discard it, in your garden compost if possible. What remains is herbal oil. Store away from sunlight and heat, preferably in a dark bottle with a well-fitting lid. Label it clearly and use within one year. If the oil begins to smell "off," it is contaminated and should be discarded.

If you can't wait ten days, follow these directions: Screw on the lid, but don't fully tighten it, and place the jar upright in a pan of water or double boiler on low heat for four hours. When the oil has the color and aroma of the herb, strain it through a fine filter, cheesecloth, or unbleached muslin. Avoid overheating, or the finished herbal oil will smell burnt, even rancid—not an incentive to use it.

If you want to turn herbal oil into a salve, do the following:

Return the oil to a clean, dry saucepan. Add 1 tablespoon coconut butter or cocoa butter per quarter cup of oil, and warm the mixture over low heat until dissolved. Pour into a clean, dry jar with a well-fitting lid, and label. If combination is too soupy for convenient vaginal application, add more coconut or cocoa butter, or reheat the mixture and melt in one or more walnut-size pieces of beeswax to adjust the solidity of the salve. To test the consistency until it's right, insert a spoon in the mixture, place the spoon in the refrigerator for five minutes, then check the hardness of the salve. The salve's consistency does not lessen the therapeutic benefits of the herbal oil, so prepare it according to your individual preference. Whenever you handle salve, use a teaspoon, not your fingers, to minimize contamination.

While some herb salves are multipurpose, note that any oil-based preparation is not ideal when yeast or fungal infections are present because these life forms thrive in moist, hot environments, and salves helps keep warmth and moisture in tissues. In these situations, use herb tinctures or extracts because the alcohol helps dry the fungal infection.

St. John's wort oil should be a red color and acts as an anti-inflammatory lubricant. Calendula oil should be golden and is especially good for healing small tears or abrasions in vaginal mucosa. Both are antiviral, though the extent of their effectiveness is variable. Wild yam oil is the basis for many natural creams used specifically in menopause because it improves vaginal lubrication and reduces inflammation. In addition, its plant sterols may be absorbed, promoting local tissue changes or systemic health effects. It is not proven that wild yam salves promote hormonal balance (though the herb taken as tea or extract does have proven hormonal effects on stress and inflammation, at least). Comfrey has no warnings or cautions when used vaginally for moistening dry mucous membranes; in fact, nothing is better for thin, inflamed, or raw surfaces.

How to Make Your Own Menopause Formula

If you would like to create an herbal formula that addresses your particular menopause health concerns, the guidelines below can help you make sense of the kaleidoscope of healing plants from which to choose.

Identifying Health Challenges

- If possible, ask women relatives, especially your mother, about their own experiences with menopause. See if you can discern any patterns in your family's history.
- List your most important health challenges.

Sadly, many of the mothers, older aunts, and even grandmothers of women entering menopause today had hysterectomies at an early age, so there is no natural history of menopause from which to learn. Even if that is true in your family, take a quiet ten minutes to write your most important health challenges on a sheet of paper. Identify your single most important concern. If you describe your top priority in more than a few words ("crippling hot flashes" or "risk of osteoporosis"), try to be more concise. After you list your top priority, add a short list of additional health concerns that mean a lot to you.

As you rate the seriousness of your health concerns, be honest with yourself. Your list is just for your eyes, for your judgment, for your health. For example: "Hot flashes are making me crazy; my mood swings would sort out if I could just get some sleep." Identifying sleep as a priority will help you decide which herbs to choose at the next stage of creating your personal formula.

Or, perhaps, "Hot flashes? Not a problem. Only had night sweats twice all year, after late-night coffee and great Mexican food. Eat right most of the time; no risk factors other than normal aging—no deep worries about my heart. Irregular cycle is a major problem—might get pregnant in my new relationship, and that would be hard on me." The major challenge here is to regulate menstrual cycles.

Setting Health Goals

To get a complete picture of your state of health, compare your list of challenges to the items listed in the accompanying box. Which items are on both lists? Those are the ones that probably need the most attention.

- After you identify what bothers you most, restate your problems as goals—the positive state of health you wish to achieve.

Redefining problems as positive goals is the best way to find out what you really want for yourself. For example, the problem of irritability might be expressed as a deep desire for tranquillity. On a practical level, this step helps you recognize the health properties, or actions, of herbs that will take you where you want to go.

Choosing Herbs

- Jot down one or two possible herbs for each of your most important areas of concern. While reading this book, have certain herbs seemed appropriate for meeting your needs? If so, list them in the appropriate category. If an herb appears more than once, it is probably a "keeper" for your customized formula.

Here are some guidelines for choosing herbs:

- Name just five to seven herbs, each with the greatest "bouquet" of herbal properties or actions you want. Concentrate on those meeting your greatest concern and needs.
- Check the dosage levels of your choices; note suggested combinations and cautions listed in the "Materia Medica."
- Keep any strong herbs (see the "Materia Medica" to determine which are strong) at the bottom of your list. Use smaller proportions of strong or really strong- tasting herbs.
- Put one herb with the largest number of actions that are important to you at the top of your list; use twice as much of it as the others.

Your most important herb will probably be a tonic, which can be used safely long term and in liberal amounts. Strong herbs are meant to be used in small doses.

Seven Overlapping Areas of Concern for Menopausal Women

1. Hot flashes (cardiovascular system)
2. Osteoporosis (musculoskeletal system)
3. Vaginal dryness or atrophy, which may lead to increased incidence of cystitis (reproductive and urinary systems)
4. Irregular cycle and spotting (reproductive system)
5. Increased cardiovascular risk in proportion to low estrogen (reproductive and cardiovascular systems)
6. Pain and dysmenorrhea with characteristic "dragging" sensations (nervous and reproductive systems)
7. Links between arthritic changes with age, pain threshold, and depression (nervous system and musculoskeletal system)

Let's say you have listed all the herbs that meet your special concerns. This is not yet a formula. In fact, your list may include more than seven herbs, and all your body systems may seem to need help! Take a deep breath and relax. If you leave all the herbs on your long list in the final formula because they sound *soooo* nice, you may not see a clear benefit in your health. Narrow down the list to one nutritive tonic that can help more than one body system. Keep one herb for emotional equilibrium. Choose only *one* specific herb to answer your body's most urgent symptoms. Use at least 2 ounces of this main herb, and 1 ounce of each of the four to six "helper" herbs. You may, of course, have fewer than five to seven herbs in your formula.

If you have selected more than two or three herbs, consider your choices in light of three criteria: your constitution, nutrition, and state of mind. This approach, explained below, was described by herbalist Billie Potts in her book *Witches Heal.*

Constitution: Choose the preventive herbs that will do the most good today and tomorrow. What chronic problems need help? Pick the herbs with an affinity for toning the body system where these chronic problems occur. You can pick tonic herbs that also have specific benefit for menopausal issues. When we build up health in weak areas, our self-healing capacity can focus on the main one. In this way, we may use digestive tonics, even if nothing terribly "wrong" is occurring in the digestive system at the time. Herbs treat what is right as well as what is wrong, to make a stronger whole woman.

Nutrition: What nourishing herbs will support the primary herb in other body systems? In answering this question, keep two factors in mind: First, your helper herbs will work even better if they are also known to help the primary symptom causing distress. For example, motherwort reduces the primary symptom of hot flashes, and it helps nourish the nerves, liver, and reproductive system as a whole, plus it can lower high blood pressure. Second, avoid use of exotics or expensive herbs grown remotely, trying to choose herbs that both meet your needs and are available in your local environment. By doing so, you support your own bioregion and local growers. Obtaining our nutrition locally enriches the global plant community, making the planet that much more whole.

State of mind: Choose an herb that reduces stress and relaxes muscles, which in turn may help circulation. The nervines tone or improve the nerves, antispasmodics relax muscles, and analgesics or anodynes relieve pain. This group of herbs includes skullcap, passion flower, wild oats, motherwort, and valerian.

Preparing the Final Mix

If you haven't already chosen a general reproductive tonic, consider these examples: raspberry leaf *(Rubus idaeus)*, yarrow *(Achillea millefolium)*, and lady's mantle *(Alchemilla vulgaris)*. Does your formula need one or more of these in addition to the others you have selected? If one herb helps all the areas, great. If one herb covers two out of three health concerns, good job. If you just love three herbs because of earlier experience with them or their descriptions ring a bell, go with them. Now you're ready to combine your choices.

Mix the hard pieces (roots, bark, seeds, berries) in a paper bag or bowl. In a separate container combine all the lighter pieces (flowers, leaves, powders). If any of the "hard" herbs work by virtue of their smell (valerian root, cinnamon bark, fennel seeds), add them to the light herb material, first breaking up any large pieces.

Steep, or infuse, the light herbs in just-boiled water, covered with a lid, for five to thirty minutes. The longer they sit, the stronger they get. More than a half hour is not helpful, though, because volatile properties evaporate away and bitters and tannins intensify. The harder herbs don't give up their medicinal properties so easily. Simmer bark, roots, and other dense herb bits in water for ten to forty-five minutes (an average of twenty minutes), covered with a lid. If you wish, you can first simmer the hard pieces in the total amount of water; then turn off the heat and add the light pieces to the same pot. Let steep for another five to thirty minutes (usually fifteen), the time depending on the strength your taste buds will tolerate, and strain. The usual range of tea dose is 1/2 to 1 cup of tea two or three times a day. You can increase the dosage for stronger short-term effects (two to seven days).

Congratulations—you have blended your own herbal tea! The effort you have put into creating it will repay you a hundredfold in natural healing consistent with your own special needs.

Appendix C

Herbal Home Medicine Chest

Most minor health problems can be handled with a few dried herbs for teas, a few tinctures, or other compounds, such as external herb salves. The twenty-one herbs listed below provide tried-and-true relief for simple maladies. Each can be used for a few different things. All are readily available, are safe when used as described in this book, and are excellent candidates for a first home medicine chest.

If you prefer another herb that performs the same action as one on the list, you can, of course, use it instead. By all means, customize your medicine chest as needed—for example, you may want to substitute herbs that grow abundantly in your vicinity or that are effective for the most common problems that recur in your household. The important thing is to not get too many herbs in the house at once so you can learn about the ones you have and more readily maintain a fresh supply. Once you get to know the herbs in your home medicine chest, you'll find that they're as terrific as they sound.

Note that glycerin-based tinctures are occasionally recommended in the list to avoid alcohol, to provide a more pleasant taste, or to improve the herb's beneficial effect; however, it really doesn't matter if you prefer to use tinctures, glycerin-based tinctures, capsules, or tablets. Follow dosages given on product labels or recommendations in the "Materia Medica" section earlier in this book.

Herb	Actions	Uses
Chasteberry seed, tincture	Emmenagogue Hormonal normalizer	For late period For irregular cycle
Comfrey root and leaf, dried, for external compresses and poultices	Vulnerary	For superficial wounds or deep bruises
Cramp bark, tincture	Antispasmodic	For cramps
Dandelion leaf and root, for tea; or fresh leaves in spring, juiced	Diuretic	For water retention
Fennel, dried seed, for tea	Carminative	For gas
Garlic, as food or in deodorized capsules	Antimicrobial	For poor immune response

Herb	Actions	Uses
Hawthorn flower, leaf, and berry, for tea; or tincturel; also berry jam	Heart tonic	For weakness of the heart
Lavender, essential oil, externally	Antidepressant aromatherapy	For immediate relief
	Antiseptic	For a wound or an infection of the skin
Marshmallow, dried other root, for tea or syrup	Demulcent	For irritation with symptoms, inside or out
Nettle, dried, for tea and syrup	Tonic	If you seem to need everything all at once
Peppermint, dried, for tea	Antacid	For bicarbonates
Raspberry leaf, dried, for tea	Uterine tonic	For pregnancy or a need to heal the womb
Sarsaparilla, tea or tincture	Alterative	For chronic hormonal, lymph, or skin problem
Siberian ginseng, tincture	Adaptogen	For energy, endurance, or coping with stress
Skullcap, tincture	Nervine relaxant	For tension headache
St. John's wort, tincture	Antidepressant	If you have eight weeks or more to uplift mood
Valerian, glycerin tincture	Analgesic	For pain
	Hypnotic	For insomnia
Wild oats, tincture	Nervine tonic	For nervous exhaustion
Wild yam, glycerin tincture	Anti-inflammatory	For inflammation
Yarrow, dried flower, for tea	Astringent	For diarrhea, discharge, or blood loss
	Bitter	For poor digestion
Yellow dock, dried root, for tea; or glycerin tincture	Aperient, laxative	For constipation

Resources

Many of the companies listed below were started by herbalists who also teach classes and offer a wide variety of health services. Please contact them directly for brochures, catalogs, price lists, and additional information. For more complete listings than space permits here, contact the American Herbalists Association, the American Herbalists Guild, and the *Herbal Green Pages,* all of which are included below. You can also contact these organizations for referrals to herbalists, naturopaths, acupuncturists, and other natural health-care providers in your area.

The Herbal Green Pages
P.O. Box 245
Silver Spring, MD 17575
(717) 393-3295
This phone book is one of the most complete resources for products and publications.

Mail-Order Herb Companies

Adaptations
P.O. Box 1070
Captain Cook, HI 96704
(808) 328-9044
Tropical, high-quality herbs, available wholesale and retail; customer pays for shipping from Hawaii.

Avena Botanicals
219 Mill Street
Rockport, ME 04856
(207) 594-0694
Woman-owned and -operated herbal apothecary offering organic teas and a wide assortment of products.

Bisbee Botanicals
P.O. Box 218
Gila, NM 88038
(505) 535-4352
Single herb extracts, oils; specializes in ecologically gathered southwestern plants.

Blessed Herbs, Inc.
109 Barre Plains Road
Oakham, MA 01068
(800) 489-4372
Huge range of common and uncommon herb products.

Earth's Harvest, Inc.
14385 S.E. Lusted Road
Sandy, OR 97055
(503) 668-4120
Herbal salves, douche concentrates, and more.

Eclectic Institute, Inc.
14385 S.E. Lusted Road
Sandy, OR 97055
(503) 668-4120
Freeze-dried herbs in capsules, organic herb products.

Herbalist & Alchemist
P.O. Box 553
Broadway, NJ 08808
(908) 689-9020
Traditional Chinese, Native American, Western herbs and books.

HerbPharm
P.O. Box 116
Williams, OR 97544
(503) 846-7178
Organic, wild-crafted extracts, combinations, oils; also books.

Island Herbs
P.O. Box 25
Waldron Island, WA 98297-0025
The best dried red clover, nettles, kelp, edible seaweeds; many other organic, dried medicinal herbs. Send self-addressed, stamped envelope for mail-order catalog.

Montana Botanicals
P.O. Box 1365
Hamilton, MT 59840
(406) 363-6683
Ecologically gathered prairie and mountain herbs; many products.

Oak Valley Herb Farm
14648 Pear Tree Lane
Nevada City, CA 95959
(916) 265-9552
Excellent-quality dried herbs and essential oils; books.

Unitea Herbs
P.O. Box 8005, Suite 318
Boulder, CO 80306-8005
(303) 443-1248
Delicious tea blends for pleasure and for hard-bitten coffee fans and herb skeptics.

Companies Offering Mail-Order Wholesale or Bulk Herbs

(Minimum one pound each herb; other restrictions may apply.)

Blackmores, Ltd.
16 Parkside Drive
North Brunswick, NJ 08902-1218
(800) 433-9272

Pacific Botanicals
4350 Fish Hatchery Road
Grants Pass, OR 97527
(503) 479-7777

Trinity Herbs
P.O. Box 199
Bodega, CA 94922
(707) 874-3418

South American Medicinal Herbs (in Bulk)

Nattrop/New World Enterprises
530 E. 8th Street, Suite 204
Oakland, CA 94606-2825
(510) 451-7862
Environmentally conscious company; hard-to-find Brazilian herbs.

Essential Oils

Earth Essentials
6849 Filbert Avenue
Orangevale, CA 95662
(916) 988-4471
Exquisite Ayurvedic and European essential oils, blends.

Oak Valley Herb Farm
14648 Pear Tree Lane
Nevada City, CA 95959
(916) 268-3002
Most affordable, pure essential oils available by mail order.

Oshadhi
15 Monarch Bay Plaza, Suite 346
Monarch Beach, CA 92629
(800) 933-1008
Large range of retail, wholesale essential oils.

Flower Remedies

Flower Essence Services
P.O. Box 1769
Nevada City, CA 95959
(916) 265-0258
Sells flower essences and books; offers classes.

Perelandra Ltd.
P.O. Box 3603
Warrenton, VA 20188
(540) 937-2153
Sells flower essences and books.

Herb Organizations

American Botanical Council
P.O. Box 201660
Austin, TX 78720
(512) 331-1924
Publishes *HerbalGram* magazine, textbooks on herbal medicine, and scientific herb studies.

American Herbalists Association
P.O. Box 16733
Nevada City, CA 95959
Membership offers many benefits, including the best practical, low-cost clinical herbalism newsletter. Write for information.

American Herbalists Guild
P.O. Box 746555
Arvada, CO 80006-6555
(303) 423-8800
The guild's directory of herbal education programs is the most complete listing of educational programs available to date. Categorized by state; includes residential and correspondence programs; specifies programs' focus (e.g., Western). Also lists publications, computer networks, and events. The membership directory provides referrals to practicing professional herbalists.

American Holistic Health Association
P.O. Box 17400
Anaheim, CA 92817-7400
(714) 779-6152
Call for information and referrals.

The European Herbal Practitioners Alliance
Midsummer Cottage Clinic
Nether Westcote
Kingham, Oxfordshire OX7 6SD
England
Represents professional organizations of herbal practitioners throughout Europe.

Herb Research Foundation
1007 Pearl Street
Boulder, CO 80302
(303) 449-2265
Literature searches, answers to herb questions from a scientific perspective.

The International Organization of Traditional and Medical Practitioners and Researchers (IOTMPR)
P.O. Box 27555
San Francisco, CA 94127
Newsletter, education on African herbal traditions, seminars, books. Write for information; enclose $3.

Klickitat Herbalists Guild
1549 W. Jewett
White Salmon, WA 98672
(509) 493-2626
Classes, newsletter, social programs.

National Herbalists Association of Australia
3 Smail Street, Suite 305
Broadway, New South Wales 2007
Australia
(02) 211 6437
Professional organization of herbalists offers referrals in Australia, conferences. Publishes *Australian Journal of Medical Herbalism*.

The National Institute of Medical Herbalists
56 Longbrook Street
Exeter, Devon EX4 6AH
England
(01392) 426022
Britain's professional herbalists' organization; offers information on training, referrals in United Kingdom, books by members.

Northeast Herbalists Association
P.O. Box 146
Marshfield, VT 05658
(802) 456-1402
The association's membership directory provides referrals to herbalists and companies offering herb products.

Ontario Herbalists Association
11 Winthrop Place
Stoney Creek
Ontario L8G 3M3
Canada
(905) 664-6715
Publishes *Canadian Journal of Herbalism*.

Rocky Mountain Herbalist Coalition
412 Boulder Street
Boulder, CO 80302
Write for information on practitioners, gathering herbs with environmental sensitivity, classes.

The Traditional Medicines Department
World Health Organization
Geneva, Switzerland
Organizes conferences, global networking on use of herbal medicines.

United Plant Savers
P.O. Box 420
East Barre, VT 05649
A nonprofit organization for replanting and protecting endangered plants, including medicinal herbs threatened by development.

Herbal Education on Audio/Video Tape

Creative Seminars
P.O. Box 203
West Hurley, NY 12491
(914) 679-6885
Taped seminars on herbs, nutrition, and natural health.

The New Mexico Herbal Treatment Center
Tieraona Low Dog, M.D., Director
120 Aliso SE
Albuquerque, NM 87108
(505) 265-0795
Videos on foundations of herbalism, herbal pharmacology, and medicine making.

Sounds True Recording
735 Walnut Street
Boulder, CO 80302
(303) 449-6229

Herbal Education by Correspondence

American Botanical Council
P.O. Box 201660
Austin, TX 78720-1660
(512) 331-8868

SAGE
Rosemary Gladstar
P.O. Box 420
East Barre, VT 05649
(802) 479-9825

Wise Woman Center
Susun Weed
P.O. Box 64
Woodstock, NY 12498
(914) 246-8081

Residential Herbal Education

Blazing Star Herbal School
Gail Ulrich, Director
P.O. Box 6
Shelburne Falls, MA 01370
(413) 625-6875

Coastal Mountain College of Healing Arts, Inc.
1745 West 4th Avenue
Vancouver BC V6J 1M2
Canada
(403) 734-4596

Green Terrestrials
Pam Montgomery, Director
P.O. Box 266
Milton, NY 12547
(914) 795-5238

The National College of Phytotherapy
Tieraona Low Dog, M.D.
Amanda McQuade Crawford, D.Phyt., MNIMH
120 Aliso SE
Albuquerque, NM 87108
(505) 265-0795

The Rocky Mountain Center for Botanical Studies
Feather Jones, Director
P.O. Box 19254
Boulder, CO 80308-2254
(303) 442-6861

The School of Phytotherapy
Mr. Hein Zeylstra, MNIMH, Dean
The Registrar
Bucksteep Manor
Bodle Street Green
Hailsham, East Sussex BN27 4RJ
England
(0323) 833812/4

The Self-Heal School of Herbal Studies & Healing
P.O. Box 70131
San Diego, CA 92167
(619) 224-1268

The Southwest School of Botanic Medicine
Michael Moore, Director
122 Tulane SE
Albuquerque, NM 87106
(505) 255-9215

Waikato Centre for Herbal Studies
Isla Burgess, Director
P.O. Box 439
Cambridge, New Zealand
(07) 8277181

Herbal Newsletters and Journals—United States

American Herb Association (AHA) Quarterly Newsletter
P.O. Box 353
Rescue, CA 95672

Foster's Botanical and Herb Reviews
P.O. Box 106
Eureka Springs, AR 72632

HerbalGram
P.O. Box 12006
Austin, TX 78711

The Herbalist
Newsletter of the American Herbalists Guild
P.O. Box 1683
Soquel, CA 95073

Medical Herbalism
P.O. Box 33080
Portland, OR 97233

Medical Nutrition
P.O. Box 1729
Gig Harbor, WA 98335

World Research News
15300 Ventura Boulevard, Suite 405
Sherman Oaks, CA 91403

Herbal Newsletters and Journals—International

The Australian Journal of Medical Herbalism
Box 65
Kingsgrove, New South Wales 2208
Australia

The British Journal of Phytotherapy
3 King's Mill Way
Hermitage Lane, Mansfield
Notts NG18 5ER
England

Canadian Herbal Practitioners Newsletter
302-1220 Kensington Road NW
Calgary, Alberta
Canada T2N 3P5

Herbal Thymes
7 Dangar Road
Singleton, 2330
Australia

Planta Medica
Thieme Medical Publishers
381 Park Avenue South
New York, NY 10016

Other Important Addresses

Izard Ozark Natives
Steven Foster
P.O. Box 1343
Fayetteville, AR 72702
(501) 521-5887
Books, field identification guides, and herb seeds.

The National Institutes of Health
Office of Alternative Medicine
6120 Executive Plaza South, Room 450
Rockville, MD 20092-9904
(301) 402-2466
Information on research into traditional medicines using plants and other natural therapies.

Bibliography

Abraham, G. E. "Nutritional Factors in the Etiology of PMS." *Journal of Reproductive Medicine* 28, no. 7 (1983): 446–64.

Ally, M. M. "The Pharmacological Action of *Zingiber officinale*," in *Proceedings of the 4th Pan Indian Ocean Scientific Congress,* Karachi, Pakistan, Section G, 11–12, 1960.

Amann, W. "Improvement of *Acne vulgaris* with *Agnus castus* (Agnolyt)." *Ther. d. Gegenw.* 106: 124–6.

Asimov, Isaac. *The Human Body.* New York: Mentor, 1963.

Barnes, S., and T. G. Peterson. "Biochemical Targets of the Isoflavone Genistein in Tumor Cell Lines." *Proceedings of the Society for Experimental Biology and Medicine* 208, no. 1 (1995): 10–38.

Barnhart, Edward, pub. *Physician's Desk Reference*, 1992. Oradell, N.J.: Medical Economics Data, 1992.

Beckham, Nancy, N.D. "Phyto-oestrogens and Compounds That Affect Oestrogen Metabolism." *Australian Journal of Medical Herbalism* 7, no. 1 (1995): 11–16; no. 2 (1995): 27–33.

Bergner, Paul, ed. "Chaste-Tree *(Vitex agnus-castus)*." *Medical Herbalism* 2, no. 5 (1990): 1, 6.

Berkow, Robert, et al. *Merck Manual*, 15th ed. Rahway, N.J.: Merck & Co., 1987.

Bianchi, G., et al. "Effects of Gonadotrophin-releasing Hormone Agonist on Uterine Fibroids and Bone Density." *Maturitas* 11 (1989): 179–85.

Colbin, Annemarie, *Food and Healing.* New York: Ballantine, 1986.

"Consensus Statement on Progestin Use in Postmenopausal Women." Editorial. *Maturitas* 11 (1988): 175–77.

Culbreth, David, M.D. *Manual of Materia Medica and Pharmacology.* Sandy, Oreg.: Eclectic Institute, 1927.

Dentali, S. "Hormones and Yams." *American Herb Association Quarterly Newsletter* 10, no. 4 (1994).

Ellingwood, R. *American Materia Medica, Therapeutics and Pharmacognosy.* Portland, Oreg.: Eclectic Medical Pubs., 1983.

Evans, F. J., Dr., ed. *British Herbal Pharmacopoeia.* Bournemouth, U.K.: Megaron Press, 1983.

Felter, H. W. *The Eclectic Materia Medica, Pharmacology and Therapeutics.* 1922. Reprint, Portland, Oreg.: Eclectic Medical Pubs., 1983.

Felter, H. W., and J. U. Lloyd. *King's American Dispensatory,* 18th ed. 2 vols. 1898. Sandy, Oreg.: Eclectic Medical Pubs., 1983.

Foster, Steven, and James Duke. *Eastern/Central Medicinal Plants.* Peterson Field Guide Series. Boston: Houghton Mifflin, 1990.

Gaby, Alan, M.D. "Multi-level Yam Scam." *American Herb Association Quarterly Newsletter* 12, no. 1 (1996).

Garland, Sarah. *The Herb Garden.* New York: Penguin, 1984.

Grieves, Maud. *Modern Herbal.* New York: Dover, 1933.

Gunn, J. D. *New Domestic Physician or Home Book of Health.* N.p.: Moore, Wilstach & Keys, 1861.

Hahn G., et al. "Monchspfeffer (Monkspepper)." *Notabene Medici* 16 (1986): 233–6, 297–301.

Hobbs, Christopher. "Vitex: The Female Herb." *The American Herb Association Quarterly Newsletter* VII, no. 3 (1990): 5.

Hoerhammer, L., et al. "Chemistry, Pharmacology, and Pharmaceutics of the Components from *Viburnum prunifolium* and *V. opulus.*" *Botanical Magazine* (Tokyo) 79 (1966): 510–25.

Horrobin, D. F. "The Role of Essential Fatty Acids and Prostaglandins in the Premenstrual Syndrome." *Journal of Reproductive Medicine* 28, no. 7 (1983): 465–8.

Jarboe, C. H., et al. "Uterine Relaxant Properties of Viburnum." *Nature* 212, no. 5064 (1966), 837.

Kaptchuk, Ted. *The Web That Has No Weaver.* New York: Congdon & Weed, 1983.

Kayser, H. W., and S. Istanbyulluoglu. "Treatment of PMS Without Hormones." *Hippokrates* 25, no. 25: 717.

Keville, Kathi. *Illustrated Herb Encyclopedia.* New York: Mallard, 1991.

_____, ed. "GLA Studies." *American Herb Association Quarterly Newsletter* 4, no. 4 (1986): 16.

_____, ed. "Menopausal Herbs." *American Herb Association Quarterly Newsletter* 11, no. 3 (1995).

Kubota, S., and S. Nakashima. "The Study of *Leonurus sibericus L. ii.* Pharmacological Study of the Alkaloid 'Leonurin' Isolated from *Leonurus sibericus L.*" *Folia Pharmacologica Japonica* 11, no. 2 (1930): 159–67.

Kuroda, K., and T. Kaku. "Pharmacological and Chemical Studies on the Alcohol Extract of *Capsella bursa-pastoris.*" *Life Sciences* 8, no. 3 (1969): 151–5.

Kuroda, K., and K. Takagi. "Physiologically Active Substances in *Capsella bursa-pastoris.*" *Nature* 220, no. 5168 (1968): 707–8.

Lee, John. R., M.D. "Osteoporosis Reversal: The Role of Progesterone." *International Clinical Nutrition Review* 10, no. 3 (199): 384–91.

Lutomski, J. "Chemistry and the Therapeutic Use of Licorice *(Glycyrrhiza glabra L.)." Pharmazie in Unserer Zeit* 12, no. 2 (1983): 49–54.

Mabey, Richard, ed. *The New Age Herbalist*. New York: Macmillan, Collier, 1988.

McIntyre, Anne. *Herbs for Common Ailments*. New York: Simon & Schuster, Element Books, 1992.

McQuade Crawford, Amanda. "Menopause—Graceful Rite of Change." *Essays on Herbalism,* vol. 2. Edited by Michael Tierra. Englewood Cliffs, N.J.: Prentice Hall, in press.

_____."The Role of Phytosterols in Women's Health." Symposium lecture, Breitenbush Herb Retreat, Breitenbush, Oreg., 1989.

Mills, Simon, M.A., MNIMH. *The Dictionary of Modern Herbalism—A Comprehensive Guide to Practical Herbal Therapy*. Rochester, Vt.: Healing Arts Press, 1988.

Moore, Michael. *Medicinal Plants of the Desert and Canyon West*. Santa Fe: Museum of New Mexico Press, 1989.

_____. *Medicinal Plants of the Mountain West*. Santa Fe: Museum of New Mexico Press, 1979.

_____. *Medicinal Plants of the Pacific West*. Santa Fe: Red Crane Books, 1993.

Moore, Michael, and Daniel Gagnon. *Clinical Herbal Repertory*. Self-published, 1986.

Mowrey, Daniel. *The Scientific Validation of Herbal Medicine*. N.p.: Cormorant Books, 1986.

Murray, M., and J. Pizzorno. *Encyclopedia of Natural Medicine*. Rocklin, Calif.: Prima, 1990.

Northrup, Christiane, M.D. *Women's Bodies, Women's Wisdom*. New York: Bantam Books, 1994.

Notelovitz, Morris, M.D., and Marsha Ware. *Stand Tall! Preventing Osteoporosis*. Gainesville, Fla.: Triad, 1982.

Paul, Michele. *The Women's Pharmacy*. New York: Simon & Schuster, Cornerstone Library, 1983.

Pearson, C., et al. *Taking Hormones and Women's Health—Choices, Risks and Benefits*. Washington, D.C.: National Women's Health Network, 1995.

Polyakov, N. G. *A Study of the Biological Activity of Infusions of Valerian and Motherwort and Their Mixtures*. Moscow: Information of the First All Russian Session of Pharmacists, 1964: 319–24.

Potts, Billie. *Witches Heal*. Ann Arbor, Mich.: DuReve, 1988.

Ritz, Sandra, "Growing Through Menopause." *Medical Self-Care* (Winter 1981): 70–4.

Rothenberg, Robert, M.D. *Medical Dictionary and Health Manual*. New York: Signet, 1983.

Samuels, Michael, M.D., and Nancy Samuels. *The Well Adult*. New York: Simon & Schuster, 1991.

Sharaf, A., et al. "Glycyrrhetic Acid as an Active Estrogenic Substance Separated from *Glycyrrhiza glabra* (liquorice)." *Egyptian Journal of Pharmaceutical Science* 16, no. 2 (1975): 245–51.

Shauenberg, P., and F. Paris. *Guide to Medicinal Plants*. New Canaan, Conn.: Keats, 1977.

Sloane, Ethel. *Biology of Women*, 2d ed. Albany, N.Y.: Delmar, 1985.

Smith, S. "*Vitex agnus-castus*." Pamphlet translated by the author, orig. in *Zeitschrift für Phytotherapie* (July 1986).

Tierra, Lesley. *The Herbs of Life*. Freedom, Calif.: The Crossing Press, 1992.

Tierra, Michael, ed. *Essays on Herbalism; The American Herbalists Guild*. Freedom, Calif.: The Crossing Press, 1992.

———, ed. *Planetary Herbology*. Santa Fe: Lotus Press, 1988.

Vander, A. J., and D. S. Luciano. *Human Physiology,* 5th ed. New York: McGraw-Hill, 1980.

Vogel, Virgil. *American Indian Medicine*. Norman: University of Oklahoma Press, 1970.

Weed, Susun. *Wise Woman Ways: Menopausal Years*. Woodstock, N.Y.: Ash Tree, 1992.

Weiss, R. F. *Herbal Medicine*. Beaconsfield, England: Beaconsfield, 1988.

Williams, Sue Rodwell. *Essentials of Nutrition and Diet Therapy*, 5th ed. New York: Times Mirror/Mosby, 1990.

Wood, Matthew. *The Magical Staff,* Berkeley: North Atlantic Books, 1992.

Wren, R. C. *Potter's New Cyclopedia*, 15th ed. Saffron Walden, U.K.: C. W. Daniel, 1988.

Index

The Natural Remedy Book for Women
By Diane Stein

This best-seller includes information on ten natural healing methods—vitamins and minerals, herbs, naturopathy, homeopathy and cell salts, amino acids, acupressure, aromatherapy, flower essences, gemstones and emotional healing. Remedies from all ten methods are given for fifty common health problems.
"A must-read for women."—*Booklist*
$16.95 • Paper • ISBN: 0-89594-525-8

Pocket Herbal Reference Guide
By Debra St. Clair, Master Herbalist

A user-friendly, concise introduction to the basics of herbal medicine, this handy guide is perfect for carrying along when shopping for herbs. Includes therapeutic uses of over 140 medicinal plants, natural remedies for over 100 health problems, and over 60 sample formulas.
"The remedy to help a person quit smoking may be worth the price of the book itself."
—*Canadian Journal of Herbalism*
$6.95 • Paper • ISBN: 0-89594-568-1

Pocket Guide to Aromatherapy
by Kathi Keville

Professional aromatherapists will find this guide convenient to carry, and beginners will discover a wealth of concise, easy-to-read descriptions of the most popular essential oils. A quick introduction to using this powerful form of therapy to improve quality of life.
$6.95 • Paper • ISBN: 0-89594-815-X

Pocket Guide to Naturopathic Medicine
by Judith Boice

Combining the best of contemporary medical wisdom with effective natural therapies, naturopathic medicine works with the body's innate healing capacity. Perfect for quick reference, this book offers an introduction to naturopathic philosophy and techniques as well as simple home remedies for common ailments.
$6.95 • Paper • ISBN: 0-89594-821-4

A Wisewoman's Guide to Spells, Rituals, and Goddess Lore
By Elisabeth Brooke

This remarkable guide to goddess wisdom, spells, rituals and recipes includes
such topics as:
• Goddess worship, past and present • A brief history of witchcraft • Starcraft and the moon •
Festivals and the wheel of the year • How to create rituals • Ethics in witchcraft • Spellcraft •
Developing psychic skills • Divination—the tarot • Herbal Lore
$ 12.95 • Paper • ISBN: 0-89594-779-X

Please look for these books at your local bookstore or order from
The Crossing Press
P.O. Box 1048, Freedom, CA 95019.
Add $2.50 for the first book and 50¢ for each additional book. Or call toll free 800-777-1048 with your credit card order.